Bariatric and Metabolic Surgery

Seung Ho Choi • Kazunori Kasama

Editors

Bariatric and Metabolic Surgery

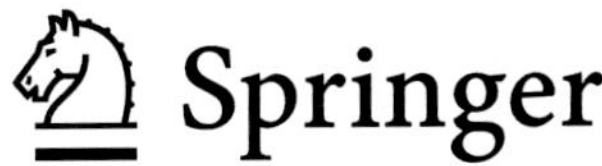 Springer

Editors
Seung Ho Choi
Department of Surgery
Gangnam Severance Hospital
Seoul
Korea

Kazunori Kasama
Weight Loss and Metabolic
Surgery Center
Yotsuya Medical Cube
Tokyo
Japan

Videos to this book can be accessed at http://www.springerimages.com/videos/978-3-642-35590-5

ISBN 978-3-662-51160-2   ISBN 978-3-642-35591-2   (eBook)
DOI 10.1007/978-3-642-35591-2
Springer Heidelberg New York Dordrecht London

Foreword

Bariatric surgery has grown exponentially in recent years detonated by the great obesity epidemic beginning in the 1970s and the advent of minimally invasive surgery in the mid-1990s. The gradual development and standardization of safer, more effective, and durable operations, such as Roux-en Y gastric bypass (RYGB), bilio-pancreatic diversion, duodenal switch, adjustable gastric banding and sleeve gastrectomy account for advances over the last decade.

Today, more than 200,000 bariatric procedures are performed each year in the United States and almost twice that figure worldwide. Since 2003 when the first bariatric surgery was performed in Korea, the annual number of cases has markedly increased. More than 1,000 bariatric procedures were done each year by laparoscopic approach.

The dramatic reduction in postoperative pain, wound complications, shorter hospital stay and operative mortality of less than 1 % are attributed to laparoscopic approach. Also Korean surgeons are familiar to the laparoscopic-assisted gastrectomy for gastric cancer, so it is not awkward for us to do various bariatric procedures.

This book, *Bariatric and Metabolic Surgery*, is intended to provide the reader with a comprehensive overview of the current status of bariatric surgery. It is our intention to address issues of interest not only technique, pre- and post-operative care, revisional surgery, metabolic effects (metabolic surgery), controversial subjects, or any other specific entities peculiar to bariatric surgery.

Bariatric and metabolic surgery is one of the most important and fascinating procedure and is a promising new field and considered it as "Blue Ocean" in Japan and Korea. This book will help you understand what the standards of care are for the field in general and for each of the operations regularly used to treat obesity and metabolic syndrome.

I hope that you encounter as much enjoyment reading this book, *"Bariatric and Metabolic Surgery"*.

Youn-Baik Choi, MD, FACS
Gangnam Severance Hospital,
Yonsei University College of Medicine

Preface

Bariatric surgery is the most important treatment modality to manage the morbid obesity and evolve to treat the metabolic disease. As the surgical tools and knowledge are developed, new surgical techniques should be established. Now, accumulation of laparoscopic surgical techniques has expanded the application of various procedures for bariatric and metabolic surgery.

First of all, it was wonderful for us to have been asked to be editors. Immediately we defined our goal for this book and authors who have extensive experience in their respective filed would be selected to compose each chapter. This book presents state of the art knowledge on bariatric and metabolic surgery. All of authors try to share and exchange their experience, which is helpful for all who are involved or interested in bariatric and metabolic surgery. We do believe that through this book, effective surgical technique will be established with enhanced safety and outcomes. Furthermore, we provide the surgical video, which all readers can access freely on the website (http://www.springerimages.com/videos/978-3-642-35590-5).

We are deeply honored to have a chance to work together with all of authors and would like to express our sincerity too for great efforts to publish this book. Also, we like to thank Ms Lauren Kim at Springer Korea, who devoted her great efforts to publish this book and Ms Ute Heilmann and Mr. Claus-Dieter Bachem for their supports at Springer.

Seung Ho Choi
Kazunori Kasama

Contents

Part III Revisional Surgery and Management of Complications

Contributors

Seung Ho Choi, MD, PhD Department of Surgery, Gangnam Severance Hospital, Yonsei University College of Medicine, Seoul, Korea

Kyung Yul Hur, MD, PhD Department of Surgery, Soonchunhyang University Hospital, Yongsan-gu, Seoul, Republic of Korea

Susumu Inamine, MD Department of Endoscopic Surgery, Nakagami General Hospital, Okinawa, Japan

Kazunori Kasama, MD, FACS Weight Loss and Metabolic Surgery Center, Yotsuya Medical Cube, Tokyo, Japan

Seong Min Kim, MD, PhD Department of Surgery, Gachon University Gil Hospital, Gachon University of Medicine and Science, Incheon, Korea

Yong Jin Kim, MD, PhD Department of Surgery, Soonchunhyang University Hospital, Yongsan-gu, Seoul, Republic of Korea

Seigo Kitano, MD Department of Gastroenterological and Pediatric Surgery, Oita University Faculty of Medicine, Oita University, Oita, Japan

Joo Ho Lee, MD Department of Surgery, Ewha Womans University School of Medicine, Seoul, Korea

Takeshi Naitoh, MD, FACS Department of Surgery, Tohoku University Hospital, Sendai, Japan

Masayuki Ohta, MD Department of Gastroenterological and Pediatric Surgery, Oita University Faculty of Medicine, Oita University, Oita, Japan

Do Joong Park, MD Department of Surgery, Seoul National University College of Medicine, Seoul, Korea

Ji Yeon Park, MD Department of Surgery, Soonchunhyang University Hospital, Yongsan-gu, Seoul, Republic of Korea

Yosuke Seki, MD Head of Obesity and Diabetes Research Unit, Weight Loss and Metabolic Surgery Center, Yotsuya Medical Cube, Tokyo, Japan

Part I

General Knowledge for Bariatric and Metabolic Surgery

Physiology of Morbid Obese Patients

1

Seung Ho Choi

1.1 Introduction

Regulations of food intake and energy expenditure are important to maintain normal weight [1]. Ghrelin produced by the stomach modulates short-term appetitive control, and leptin is produced by adipose tissue to signal fat storage reserves in the body and mediates long-term appetitive controls. For several reasons, homeostasis of energy balance can be broken, of which underlying mechanisms are remain incompletely understood. When calorie intake exceeds energy expenditure, the extra energy is stored in various organs. The main characteristic of obesity is long-term imbalance between calorie intake and energy expenditure, resulting in over accumulation of fat in body.

The main causes of obesity are excessive food intake, decreased physical activity, and genetic susceptibility. In some cases, endocrine disorders, medications, psychiatric illness, or other factors are involved.

1.2 The Source of Fat in Our Body

Most of dietary fat is in the form of triglycerides (TAG), cholesterol, and phospholipids. Among them, TAG is most important in obesity. Dietary TAG, which cannot be absorbed by the intestine, are digested into free fatty acids and monoglycerides. Once across the intestinal barrier, they are reformed into triglycerides and packaged into chylomicrons or liposomes, which are released into the blood. Finally, they are mainly captured by hepatocytes, adipocytes, or muscle fibers. TAG is the main source of energy and important components of body. However, excess TAG is accumulated in many organs.

In the postprandial state of energy excess, surplus carbohydrates are catabolized to form acetyl-CoA, which is a feedstock for the fatty acid synthesis pathway (lipogenesis) (Fig. 1.1). Taken together, excess food is stored as TCA in various organs.

1.3 Adipose Tissue

Adipose is a dynamic tissue which interacts with other organs and has important endocrine functions [2]. The major form of adipose tissue is white adipose tissue, WAT. White adipose cells (or white adipocytes) store and release energy in the form of lipids (mainly triglycerides) [3]. We can

S.H. Choi, MD, PhD
Department of Surgery, Gangnam Severance Hospital, Yonsei University College of Medicine, 211 Eonju-ro, Gangnam-gu, 135-720 Seoul, Korea
e-mail: choish@yuhs.ac

S.H. Choi, K. Kasama (eds.), *Bariatric and Metabolic Surgery*,
DOI 10.1007/978-3-642-35591-2_1, © Springer-Verlag Berlin Heidelberg 2014

Fig. 1.1 Lipogenesis

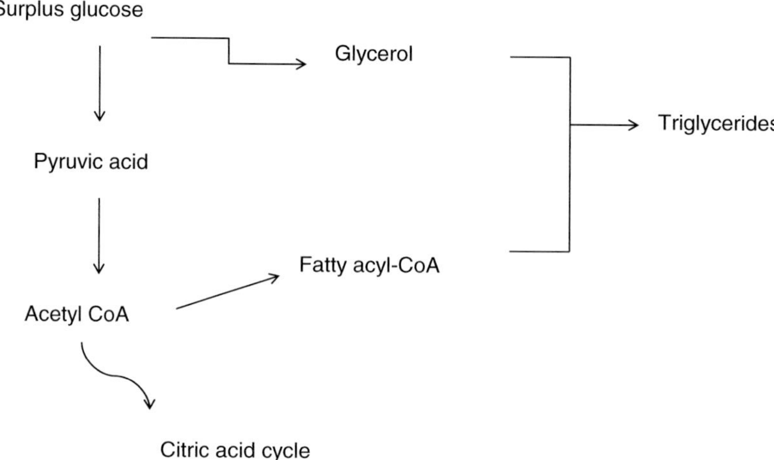

get energy from white adipose cells during fasting. Also, white adipose cells have the ability to secrete hormones and cytokines [4]. Brown adipose cells (or brown adipocytes), which are darkly pigmented due to the high density of mitochondria in cytochromes, store also triglycerides and produce heat by burning fatty acids to maintain body temperature [5]. Brown and white adipocytes are located together in the subcutaneous tissue or in the visceral peritoneum, forming a multi-depot adipose organ [6]. The main components of white adipose tissue (WAT) are white adipocytes, whereas brown adipose tissue (BAT) is mainly composed of brown adipocytes. Also, intermediate forms of adipocytes between white and brown adipocytes are present in all depots of the adipose organ [7, 8].

Under the influence of insulin, the adipocyte takes up free fatty acids (FFAs) from the blood and then stores them in the form of intracellular lipid droplets and fat mobilization is suppressed. In adipose tissue, fatty acids may be released into circulation for delivery to other tissues.

In a surplus caloric state, adipocytes become hypertrophic, which induce cellular signaling for the recruitment, proliferation, and differentiation of new fat cells. Failure of new adipogenesis may cause existing fat cells to undergo excessive hypertrophy, causing adipocyte dysfunction, which results in pathogenic adipocytes, and adipose tissue endocrine and immune responses [9, 10]. And, dysfunction of adipogenesis results in ectopic fat storage, i.e., intra-abdominal, perimuscular, perivascular, pericardial, and periosteal fat accumulation [11]. Ectopic fat storage such as pericardial and perivascular space may have direct pathogenic effects on the myocardium, coronary arteries, and peripheral vessels, via dysregulated local secretion of vasoactive and inflammatory factors [9, 12]. Also, extra lipid is accumulated in other tissues or organs such as pancreatic beta cells, liver, and skeletal muscle, leading to lipotoxicity.

In visceral obesity, the dyslipidemia is frequently observed. It includes high levels of triglycerides and low levels of high-density lipoprotein (HDL) cholesterol. Hypertriglyceridemia is associated with an increased cholesteryl ester transfer, protein-mediated transfer of TG from the TG-rich lipoprotein to LDL and HDL, and of cholesteryl ester from LDL and HDL to TG-rich lipoproteins. The resulting TG enrichment of the LDL and HDL particles are good substrates for lipolysis by hepatic lipase, an enzyme that plays a key role of HDL metabolism leading to the depletion of the lipid core of these lipoproteins, thereby forming small, dense LDL and HDL particles. Smaller HDL become more sensitive to degradation and increased clearance from the blood [13]. Apart from low level of HDL, small, dense LDL are highly atherogenic [14, 15]. As a result, dyslipidemia associated with visceral obesity is a major cardiovascular risk factor.

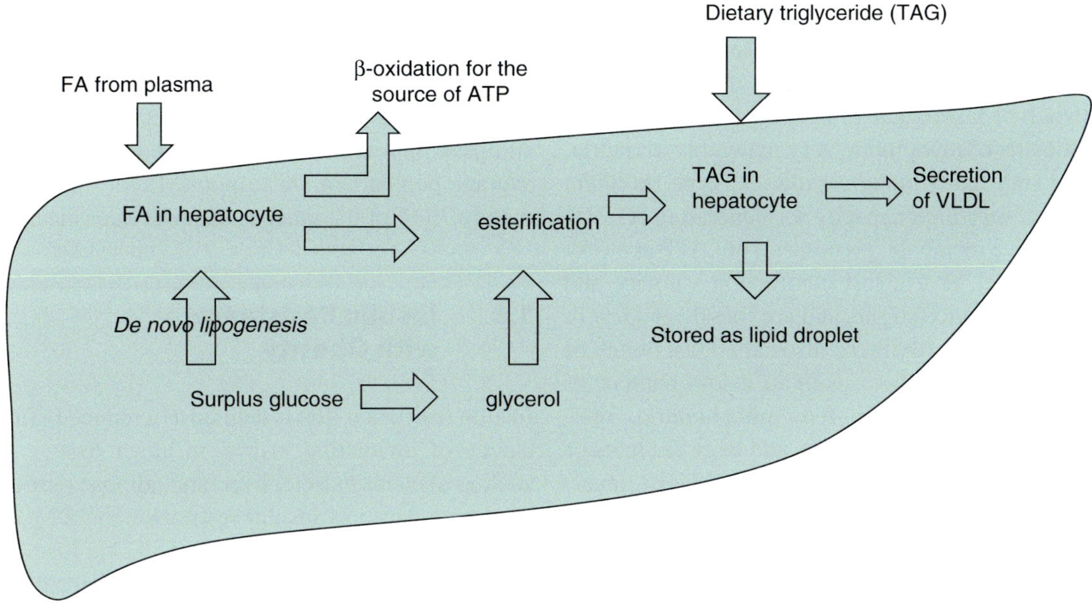

Fig. 1.2 Energy metabolism in liver. *FA* fatty acid, *TAG* triglycerides, *VLDL* very low density lipoproteins

1.4 Liver

Dietary triglycerides (TAG) are transported to the liver from intestines. In addition, hepatic TAG synthesis from fatty acids and glycerol occurs [16]. TAG from liver are secreted into blood as very low-density lipoproteins (VLDL). VDRL are either stored in adipose tissue as re-esterified TAG or metabolized into FA and used as energy source (Fig. 1.2).

The sources of FA are from either the plasma or FA newly synthesized within the liver through lipogenesis. Lipogenesis is the process of fatty acid synthesis that surplus glucose is converted into acetyl-CoA.

Hepatic TAG synthesis is stimulated by the insulin in the postprandial state. Also, insulin suppresses the secretion of VLDL and the b-oxidation of fatty acids to generate ATP. Thus, hyperinsulinemia, common phenomenon of obesity, favors overproduction of TAG in liver. Excessive TAG is accumulated as lipid droplets in hepatocytes (hepatic steatosis) and induces inflammatory and hepatocellular ballooning injury (nonalcoholic steatohepatitis), eventually leading to fibrosis and cirrhosis [17].

1.5 Muscle

Skeletal muscle constitutes 40 % of body weight in normal persons and uses 35–40 % of total oxygen consumption in the resting state. During exercise, consumption of oxygen and metabolic fuels increases markedly to provide the adenosine triphosphate (ATP) necessary for the contractile process [18]. Glycogen, glucose, and free fatty acids are main fuels for energy metabolism in muscle.

The skeletal muscle can be categorized into type I, type IIa, and type IIb. Type I and type IIa fibers appear red due to the presence of myoglobin, and type IIb fibers are white due to the absence of myoglobin. Type I fibers, also called slow twitch or slow oxidative fibers, contain large amounts of myoglobin, many mitochondria, and many blood capillaries. Type I fibers have an ability to split ATP at a slow rate, have a slow contraction velocity, very resistant to fatigue, and have a high capacity to generate ATP by oxidative metabolic processes using mainly triglycerides. Type IIa fibers, also called fast twitch or fast oxidative fibers, contain very large amounts of myoglobin, very many mitochondria, and very many blood capillaries. Type IIa fibers have a very high capacity for generating ATP by oxidative metabolic processes, split ATP at a very rapid rate, have a fast contraction velocity and are resistant to fatigue, and are found very few in humans. Type IIb fibers, also called fast twitch or fast glycolytic fibers, contain a low content of myoglobin, relatively few mitochondria, relatively few blood capillaries, and large amounts of glycogen. Type IIb fibers generate ATP by anaerobic metabolic processes, not able to supply skeletal muscle fibers continuously with sufficient ATP, fatigue easily, split ATP at a fast rate, and have a fast contraction velocity.

In obesity, the structural and metabolic changes in skeletal muscle occur. In general, obese population have a larger lean body mass than nonobese subjects [19]. In some obese people, muscle mass can be much lower than expected (sarcopenic obesity). It is characterized by fewer type I and/or more type IIb muscle fibers in obese individuals than in lean individuals. The predominance of type II fibers in severe obesity might result in low capacity of lipid oxidation and an increase in fat storage within skeletal muscle.

Glucose transport in muscles was stimulated approximately 2.5-fold by insulin from lean persons, but there was little or no stimulation of glucose transport in muscles from severely obese patients either with or without type 2 diabetes. In muscle, fatty acids are a substrate for oxidation. Fatty acid oxidation did not differ between the muscles of lean and obese individuals but was significantly reduced in severely obese individuals [20]. In contrast, glycolytic metabolism is increased. Muscle fatty acid metabolism is more sensitive to physical activity, during which fatty acid utilization from extracellular and intracellular sources may increase enormously. Adipose tissue fat mobilization increases to meet the demands of skeletal muscle during exercise. When TAG accumulates excessively in skeletal

muscle and liver, sometimes called ectopic fat deposition, then the condition of insulin resistance arises. This may reflect a lack of exercise and an excess of fat intake. Skeletal muscles comprise approximately 45 % of body mass in an average person and are responsible for approximately 75 % of the glucose disposal after meal.

1.6 Insulin Resistance with Obesity

Insulin resistance (IR) is defined as a reduced efficiency of circulating insulin in target tissues – such as skeletal muscle, liver, and adipose tissue. The main cause of insulin resistance and DM is the fat accumulation in the body [21]. Insulin resistance manifests with decrease of insulin-stimulated glucose uptake and utilization in the skeletal muscle, impaired insulin-mediated inhibition of hepatic glucose production in the liver, and a reduced ability of insulin to inhibit lipolysis in the adipose tissue (Fig. 1.3).

Subsequent high glucose level results in compensatory hyperinsulinemia. Other important conditions associated with IR include hyperuricemia, gallstones, thrombophilia, endothelial dysfunction, and polycystic ovary syndrome.

1.7 Obesity and Heart

Obesity and insulin resistance enhance lipid synthesis in hepatocytes and increase lipolysis in adipocytes, which results in increases in circulating FFAs and TGs. Also, elevated levels of insulin stimulate FFA transport into cardiomyocytes. Thus, hyperlipidemia and hyperinsulinemia together increase FFA delivery to myocytes, resulting in lipotoxicity. Hence, increasing adiposity may set the stage for cardiac dysfunction by promoting excessive myocardial FFA use and the development of lipotoxicity. However, obesity also promotes global insulin resistance, which eventually leads to chronic systemic hyperglycemia. Glucotoxicity also contributes to cardiac injury through multiple mechanisms, including direct and indirect effects of glucose on

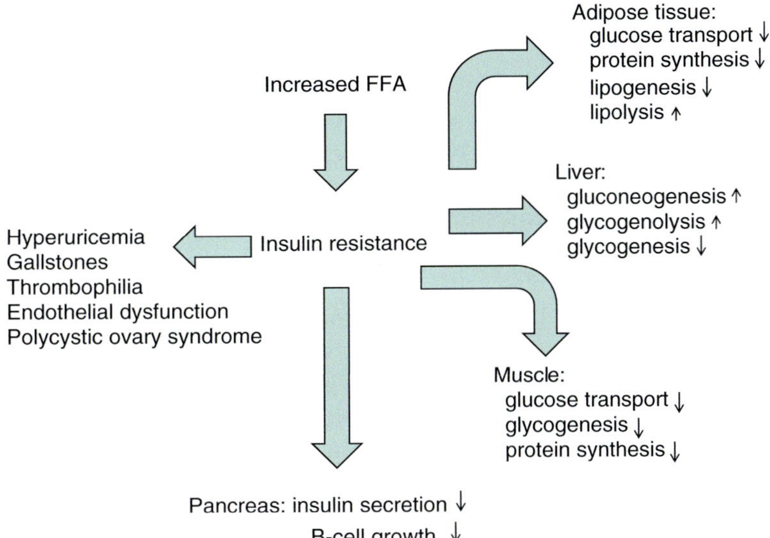

Fig. 1.3 Insulin resistance with obesity

cardiomyocytes, cardiac fibroblasts, and endothelial cells. Hyperglycemia promotes the overproduction of reactive oxygen species. In addition to lipotoxicity and glucotoxicity, atheroma in coronary artery is the most important factor in heart injury of obesity.

1.8 Obesity and Respiratory System

Obstructive sleep apnea is a common disorder with obesity and involves cessation or significant decrease in airflow in the presence of breathing effort. It is caused by obstruction of the upper airway. These episodes are associated with recurrent oxyhemoglobin desaturations and arousals from sleep. The patients may become conditioned to the daytime sleepiness and fatigue associated with significant levels of sleep disturbance. Weight loss reduces upper airway collapsibility during sleep [22].

Obstructive hypoventilation syndrome or Pickwickian syndrome is defined as the presence of awake hypercapnia (PaCO$_2$ >45 mmHg) in the obese patient (BMI >30 kg/m^2) after other causes that could account for awake hypoventilation, such as lung or neuromuscular disease, have been excluded [23]. It is distinguished from the "overlap syndrome," which is the term used to describe the association of COPD and OSA.

Malignant obesity hypoventilation syndrome (MOHS) is a subset of patients with severe OHS and characterized by severe obesity-related hypoventilation (OHS), with obstructive sleep apnea (OSA), systemic hypertension, diabetes and the metabolic syndrome, left ventricular (LV) hypertrophy with diastolic dysfunction, pulmonary hypertension, and renal and hepatic dysfunction [24]. MOHS is defined as a patient with a BMI >40 kg/m^2 with awake hypercapnia (PaCO$_2$ >45 mmHg), the metabolic syndrome, and multiorgan dysfunction related to obesity [23]. MOHS showed high mortality. The management of patients with MOHS includes short-term measures to improve the patients' medical condition and long-term measures to achieve enduring weight loss. Bariatric surgery reverses or improves the multiple metabolic and organ dysfunctions associated with MOHS [24].

1.9 Venous Thromboembolism in Obesity

Venous thromboembolism such as deep vein thrombosis or pulmonary embolism is a rare disease but can result in death, and most of those who survive suffer from serious sequel. Obesity is a proinflammatory and prothrombotic state and increases the rate of venous thromboembolism [25, 26]. Symptoms for venous thrombosis are heaviness, pain, cramps, pruritus, and paresthesia, and signs are pretibial edema, induration of the skin, hyperpigmentation, new venous ectasia, redness, pain during calf compression, and ulceration of the skin. If obese persons have any signs or symptoms of venous thrombosis, they should be checked for prevention of serious complications. The obesity induces the raised intra-abdominal pressure and decreased blood flow in the legs [27]. Also, it is postulated that obesity results in thrombosis, increased activity of the coagulation cascade, and decreased fibrinolysis [28]. In this process, elevated leptin level is strongly associated [29–31]. There may be increased inflammation, oxidative stress, and endothelial dysfunction. Also, elevated levels of lipids and glucose may contribute to the prothrombotic state [28].

Conclusion

In summary, there is consistent evidence that obesity induces a lot of different physiologic condition, compared to normal weight population. As mentioned above, the obese frequently have accompanying metabolic syndrome, including hyperinsulinemia, hypertriglyceridemia, and hypertension. Also, decreased function of the heart, lung, liver, kidney, and coagulation system is an important factor to be concerned for the management of obese patients. Understanding of physiologic condition in obesity could reduce the risk of unwanted results during the bariatric surgery.

References

1. Flier JS. Obesity wars: molecular progress confronts an expanding epidemic. Cell. 2004;116(2):337–50.
2. Scherer PE. Adipose tissue: from lipid storage compartment to endocrine organ. Diabetes. 2006;55(6): 1537–45.
3. Rosen ED, Spiegelman BM. Adipocytes as regulators of energy balance and glucose homeostasis. Nature. 2006;444(7121):847–53.
4. Friedman JM. Leptin at 14 y of age: an ongoing story. Am J Clin Nutr. 2009;89(3):973S–9.
5. Cannon B, Nedergaard J. Brown adipose tissue: function and physiological significance. Physiol Rev. 2004;84(1):277–359.
6. Cinti S. The adipose organ. Prostaglandins Leukot Essent Fatty Acids. 2005;73(1):9–15.
7. Murano I, et al. Noradrenergic parenchymal nerve fiber branching after cold acclimatisation correlates with brown adipocyte density in mouse adipose organ. J Anat. 2009;214(1):171–8.
8. Vitali A, et al. The adipose organ of obesity-prone C57BL/6J mice is composed of mixed white and brown adipocytes. J Lipid Res. 2012;53(4):619–29.
9. Capurso C, Capurso A. From excess adiposity to insulin resistance: the role of free fatty acids. Vascul Pharmacol. 2012;57(2–4):91–7.
10. Bays HE, et al. Pathogenic potential of adipose tissue and metabolic consequences of adipocyte hypertrophy and increased visceral adiposity. Expert Rev Cardiovasc Ther. 2008;6(3):343–68.
11. Pasarica M, et al. Lower total adipocyte number but no evidence for small adipocyte depletion in patients with type 2 diabetes. Diabetes Care. 2009;32(5): 900–2.
12. Gray SL, Vidal-Puig AJ. Adipose tissue expandability in the maintenance of metabolic homeostasis. Nutr Rev. 2007;65(6 Pt 2):S7–12.
13. Lamarche B, et al. Triglyceride enrichment of HDL enhances in vivo metabolic clearance of HDL apo A-I in healthy men. J Clin Invest. 1999;103(8):1191–9.
14. Taskinen MR. Diabetic dyslipidaemia: from basic research to clinical practice. Diabetologia. 2003;46(6): 733–49.
15. Verges B. Abnormal hepatic apolipoprotein B metabolism in type 2 diabetes. Atherosclerosis. 2010;211(2): 353–60.
16. Donnelly KL, et al. Sources of fatty acids stored in liver and secreted via lipoproteins in patients with nonalcoholic fatty liver disease. J Clin Invest. 2005; 115(5):1343–51.
17. Brunt EM, et al. Nonalcoholic steatohepatitis: a proposal for grading and staging the histological lesions. Am J Gastroenterol. 1999;94(9):2467–74.
18. Felig P, Wahren J. Fuel homeostasis in exercise. N Engl J Med. 1975;293(21):1078–84.

19. Forbes GB, Welle SL. Lean body mass in obesity. Int J Obes. 1983;7(2):99–107.
20. Hulver MW, et al. Skeletal muscle lipid metabolism with obesity. Am J Physiol Endocrinol Metab. 2003; 284(4):E741–7.
21. Fujioka S, et al. Contribution of intra-abdominal fat accumulation to the impairment of glucose and lipid metabolism in human obesity. Metabolism. 1987; 36(1):54–9.
22. Schwartz AR, et al. Obesity and obstructive sleep apnea: pathogenic mechanisms and therapeutic approaches. Proc Am Thorac Soc. 2008;5(2): 185–92.
23. Piper AJ, Grunstein RR. Obesity hypoventilation syndrome: mechanisms and management. Am J Respir Crit Care Med. 2011;183(3):292–8.
24. Marik PE. The malignant obesity hypoventilation syndrome (MOHS). Obes Rev. 2012;13(10): 902–9.
25. Cushman M. Epidemiology and risk factors for venous thrombosis. Semin Hematol. 2007;44(2): 62–9.
26. Ageno W, et al. Cardiovascular risk factors and venous thromboembolism: a meta-analysis. Circulation. 2008;117(1):93–102.
27. Darvall KA, et al. Obesity and thrombosis. Eur J Vasc Endovasc Surg. 2007;33(2):223–33.
28. Margaret AL, Syahruddin E, Wanandi SI. Low activity of manganese superoxide dismutase (MnSOD) in blood of lung cancer patients with smoking history: relationship to oxidative stress. Asian Pac J Cancer Prev. 2011;12(11):3049–53.
29. Dellas C, et al. Absence of leptin resistance in platelets from morbidly obese individuals may contribute to the increased thrombosis risk in obesity. Thromb Haemost. 2008;100(6):1123–9.
30. Chu NF, et al. Plasma insulin, leptin, and soluble TNF receptors levels in relation to obesity-related atherogenic and thrombogenic cardiovascular disease risk factors among men. Atherosclerosis. 2001;157(2):495–503.
31. Singh P, et al. Leptin upregulates the expression of plasminogen activator inhibitor-1 in human vascular endothelial cells. Biochem Biophys Res Commun. 2010;392(1):47–52.

Masayuki Ohta and Seigo Kitano

2.1 Introduction

Bariatric surgery has significantly decreased overall mortality and has imparted a survival advantage to patients undergoing this surgery [21], and the number of such surgeries has now rapidly increased worldwide, even in Asia [18]. Because bariatric patients usually have uncontrolled comorbidities related to obesity and psychological problems, a multidisciplinary team approach for the systematic evaluation and management of these patients is seen as an important component of a bariatric and metabolic surgery practice. In the Society of American Gastrointestinal and Endoscopic Surgeons (SAGES) guidelines, the team leader is a surgeon who must have acquired the proper education and surgical training, and other important team members include nutritionists, psychologists with specific training and experience, psychiatrists, and medical subspecialists (endocrinologists, anesthesiologists, and cardiologists, among others) [24]. The team not only preoperatively evaluates and optimizes the patients for surgery but also provides them with preoperative teaching and perioperative care. As a result, a thorough understanding of proper patient selection, appropriate preoperative evaluation, and preparation for patients and successful outcomes of bariatric and metabolic surgery can be achieved in clinical practice. This chapter reviews issues related to preoperative evaluation and preparation for bariatric surgery.

2.2 Preoperative Evaluation

2.2.1 General and Medical Evaluation

Candidates for bariatric and metabolic surgery must undergo a routine preoperative evaluation similar to the workup for other major surgeries. The aims of this evaluation are to identify current issues of comorbidities related to obesity, surgical and anesthetic risks, and nutrition and to inform and educate the patients about these issues. The evaluation list includes the following items:

- Hematological and laboratory analyses
- Chest X-ray
- Electrocardiogram
- Pulmonary function test (spirometry)
- Echocardiography
- Abdominal computed tomography
- Abdominal ultrasonography
- Polysomnography
- Upper gastrointestinal endoscopy
- Screening of *Helicobacter pylori*
- Esophageal pH monitoring and manometry (for gastric banding)

M. Ohta, MD (✉) • S. Kitano, MD
Department of Gastroenterological
and Pediatric Surgery, Oita University Faculty
of Medicine, Oita University, Oita 879-5593, Japan
e-mail: ohta@oita-u.ac.jp

S.H. Choi, K. Kasama (eds.), *Bariatric and Metabolic Surgery*,
DOI 10.1007/978-3-642-35591-2_2, © Springer-Verlag Berlin Heidelberg 2014

Hematological and laboratory analyses include a complete blood count, liver and renal function, electrolyte levels, metabolic profiles, fasting blood glucose, glycosylated hemoglobin, coagulation studies, thyroid and adrenal function, ferritin, vitamins, total iron-binding capacity, minerals, and trace elements such as iron, zinc, calcium, and magnesium. A comprehensive nutritional assessment should be performed preoperatively. The candidates frequently have deficiencies of vitamins A and D and iron [5]. These abnormalities should be corrected before the operation. Because C-peptide is a surrogate of intrinsic insulin secretion, this measurement is very important to predict remission of type 2 diabetes after bariatric and metabolic surgery [16].

Routine preoperative evaluation of left ventricular function is not recommended in noncardiac surgery [1], and transthoracic echocardiography often results in poor imaging in patients with morbid obesity. Nevertheless, preoperative assessment including echocardiography should be performed in patients with dyspnea of unknown origin, prior heart failure, and cardiomyopathy [1] and may be useful in patients with multiple obesity-related comorbidities [23]. Because decreased preoperative ejection fraction and postoperative mortality or morbidity are positively correlated [1]. Abdominal computed tomography and ultrasonography can evaluate visceral fat volume, liver size, and cholelithiasis. Hepatomegaly is cited as the most common cause to convert from a laparoscopic to an open procedure, and very low-calorie diet for 6 weeks preoperatively may be helpful to reduce liver volume and to improve access to the upper stomach when hepatomegaly is discovered [7]. Concomitant cholecystectomy for symptomatic gallbladder stones is also recommended, but prophylactic cholecystectomy for non-symptomatic gallbladder stones is still controversial [9, 25].

The anesthesiologist guidelines for patients scheduled for elective major surgery recommend considering preoperative assessment of obstructive sleep apnea with polysomnography and introducing continuous positive airway pressure [12]. Some reports recommend routine screening for obstructive sleep apnea prior to bariatric surgery [20], but the Committee of the American Society for Metabolic and Bariatric Surgery (ASMBS) does not agree with this recommendation [3].

The role of routine endoscopy for preoperative evaluation in bariatric and metabolic surgery also remains controversial. However, upper gastrointestinal endoscopy is very useful to evaluate hiatal hernia, esophagitis/gastritis, active ulcer disease, Barrett's esophagus and other lesions with a potential for malignancy, and gastrointestinal malignancies. The guidelines from the European Association for Endoscopic Surgery recommend preoperative endoscopy or radiologic evaluation with a barium meal in all bariatric patients regardless of symptoms [26]. The SAGES guidelines recommended preoperative endoscopy when suspicion of gastric pathology exists [24]. The clinical significance of routine screening for *Helicobacter pylori* has not been defined for bariatric and metabolic surgery. However, preoperative eradication therapy may be advised if this infection is present [24]. Especially in Eastern Asian countries, in which gastric cancer and *Helicobacter pylori* infection have been epidemic and the relation has been investigated [11, 30], routine upper gastrointestinal endoscopy and screening for the infection may be necessary. Because upper gastrointestinal complications including esophageal reflux and dysmotility are associated with poor outcomes after gastric banding, esophageal pH monitoring and manometry are advised in potential gastric banding candidates [9].

Preoperative screening of deep vein thrombosis to prevent pulmonary embolism using Doppler ultrasonography and D-dimer measurement has not been established in the field of bariatric surgery. However, retrievable inferior vena cava filters are effective in preventing pulmonary embolism in high-risk patients undergoing bariatric surgery who have history of venous thromboembolism [31].

2.2.2 Psychological and Behavioral Evaluation

The psychological and behavioral evaluation of candidates for bariatric and metabolic surgery is extremely important because these candidates are more likely than the overall population to have psychiatric disorders such as depression, anxiety disorder, and personality disorder [14]. These disorders may be related to poor outcome after bariatric surgery [14]. Although consensus for a standardized protocol for the psychological and behavioral evaluation is still lacking, mental health professionals evaluate the candidates using clinical interviews, symptom inventories, objective personality/psychopathology tests, and cognitive function tests [10]. Key areas to identify may include current depressive symptoms, personality disorders, trauma history, substance abuse, or purging [6]. The relatively long evaluation process with repeated visits for several months probably helps in the more precise evaluation of the candidates. Also, smoking significantly increases operative risk and the behavioral evaluation should include it [2].

Dietary counseling and education should be started preoperatively. Dietary indiscretions and maladaptive eating habits can lead to poor outcomes after bariatric surgery [28]. Postoperatively, dietary education should be reinforced because bariatric and metabolic surgery requires a lifelong change in eating habits and food choices. However, a preoperative sweet-eating behavior does not seem to be related to poor outcomes after bariatric surgery [8], and binge-eating disorder is related to better weight loss in a recent systematic review [17].

2.3 Indication and Contraindication

Recently, weight loss surgery for patients with a BMI of ≥ 35 kg/m^2 has been called "bariatric surgery" and that for patients with a BMI of <35 kg/m^2 has been termed "metabolic surgery" [15]. Presently, there is no distinct BMI cutoff value for the indication of bariatric and metabolic surgery. The indications depend on comorbidities, race, and area of the world and are described in detail in Chaps. 1, 3, 4, and 5. Given the risks of weight loss surgery, surgeons must assure themselves that patients seek this intervention and will obtain many more advantages from it compared with other strategies. Therefore, bariatric and metabolic surgery is also beneficial for elderly (>60 years) and pediatric/adolescent patients [24]. Because physical maturity is a requirement before surgery, the criteria may be limited to children over 12 years of age [22].

The SAGES guidelines state that there are no absolute contraindications to bariatric surgery [24]. Relative and clinical contraindications are as follows:

- Severe psychiatric disorder
- Severe mental retardation
- Prader-Willi syndrome
- Drug or alcohol abuse
- Cirrhosis with portal hypertension
- Active cancer
- Pregnancy

Preoperatively, the candidates should be able to comprehend the surgery, the risks involved, and the postoperative behavioral changes and lifestyle adaptation required. Bariatric and metabolic surgery can be performed in patients with mild cirrhosis without portal hypertension, but dissection around the esophagogastric junction during surgery may induce massive bleeding in patients with portal hypertension [28]. Because women should avoid pregnancy for at least 12–18 months after bariatric surgery [2], pregnancy should be included in the contraindications.

Factors that significantly increase operative risks and postoperative complications of bariatric and metabolic surgery are shown below [2, 9, 13, 19]:

- BMI >59 kg/m^2
- Age >50 years
- Congestive heart failure
- Coronary heart disease
- Stroke
- Peripheral vascular disease
- Chronic renal failure
- Chronic obstructive pulmonary disease
- Dyspnea at rest
- Smoking
- Revisional surgery

Because revisional bariatric surgery patients are at high risk of operative complications [27], another protocol is prepared for their preoperative assessment in one institution [9]. Therefore, the optimal candidates are patients who do not have any factors on the list and can fully understand the surgical process.

2.4 Preoperative Preparation

After the comprehensive evaluation by a multidisciplinary team, preoperative education and optimization including expected dietary habits, appropriate food choices, correction of nutritional abnormalities, control of obesity-related comorbidities and mental disorders, smoking cessation, and eradication of *Helicobacter pylori* should be initiated and aided by the team approach. Preoperative weight loss seems to be beneficial to decrease operation time and perioperative complications by reducing liver size and visceral fat volume, especially in super-obese patients (BMI >60 kg/m^2) [29]. However, there has been no high-level evidence of the benefit of a medical program for preoperative weight loss, especially in regard to enhancement of postoperative weight loss. ASMBS stated in their recently published position statement that a 6–12-month preoperative dietary weight loss program has not been proven to be beneficial by evidence-based reports, and the current evidence supporting preoperative weight loss only involves physician-mandated weight loss [4]. Preoperative weight loss recommended by the surgeon and/or the multidisciplinary team because of an individual patient's needs may have value for the purposes of improving surgical risk or evaluating patient adherence.

Conclusion

Candidates for bariatric and metabolic surgery are a population of high-risk patients. Good outcomes are achieved by appropriate patient selection and preparation carried out through a multidisciplinary team approach. Therefore, it is essential for the team to evaluate and educate each patient preoperatively. As well, the patients have to fully understand the procedures and the lifelong course they must commit to after surgery.

References

1. American College of Cardiology Foundation/American Heart Association Task Force on Practice Guidelines; American Society of Echocardiography; American Society of Nuclear Cardiology et al. 2009 ACCF/AHA focused update on perioperative beta blockade incorporated into the ACC/AHA 2007 guidelines on perioperative cardiovascular evaluation and care for noncardiac surgery. J Am Coll Cardiol. 2009;54:e13–118.
2. Apovian CM, Cummings S, Anderson W, et al. Best practice update for multidisciplinary care in weight loss surgery. Obesity (Silver Spring). 2009;17:871–9.
3. ASMBS Clinical Issues Committee. Peri-operative management of obstructive sleep apnea. Surg Obes Relat Dis. 2012;8:e27–32.
4. Brethauer S. ASMBS position statement on preoperative supervised weight loss requirements. Surg Obes Relat Dis. 2011;7:257–60.
5. Buchwald H, Ikramuddin S, Dorman RB, et al. Management of the metabolic/bariatric surgery patient. Am J Med. 2011;124:1099–105.
6. Collazo-Clavell ML, Clark MM, McAlpine DE, et al. Assessment and preparation of patients for bariatric surgery. Mayo Clin Proc. 2006;81:S11–7.
7. Colles SL, Dixon JB, Marks P, et al. Preoperative weight loss with a very-low-energy diet: quantitation of changes in liver and abdominal fat by serial imaging. Am J Clin Nutr. 2006;84:304–11.
8. Dixon JB, O'Brien PE. Selecting the optimal patient for LAP-BAND placement. Am J Surg. 2002;184:17S–20.
9. Eldar S, Heneghan HM, Brethauer S, et al. A focus on surgical preoperative evaluation of the bariatric patient – the Cleveland clinic protocol and review of the literature. Surgeon. 2011;9:273–7.
10. Fabricatore AN, Crerand CE, Wadden TA, et al. How do mental health professionals evaluate candidates for bariatric surgery? Survey results. Obes Surg. 2006;16:567–73.
11. Fukase K, Kato M, Kikuchi S, et al. Effect of eradication of *Helicobacter pylori* on incidence of metachronous gastric carcinoma after endoscopic resection of early gastric cancer: an open-label, randomised controlled trial. Lancet. 2008;372:392–7.
12. Gross JB, Bachenberg KL, Benumof JL, et al. Practice guidelines for the perioperative management of patients with obstructive sleep apnea: a report by the American Society of Anesthesiologists Task Force on Perioperative Management of patients with obstructive sleep apnea. Anesthesiology. 2006;104:1081–93.
13. Gupta PK, Gupta H, Kaushik M, et al. Predictors of pulmonary complications after bariatric surgery. Surg Obes Relat Dis. 2012;8:574–81.
14. Kinzl JF, Schrattenecker M, Traweger C, et al. Psychosocial predictors of weight loss after bariatric surgery. Obes Surg. 2006;16:1609–14.

15. Lakdawala M, Bhasker A. Report: Asian consensus meeting on metabolic surgery. Recommendations for the use of bariatric and gastrointestinal metabolic surgery for treatment of obesity and type II diabetes mellitus in the Asian population: August 9th and 10th, 2008, Trivandrum, India. Obes Surg. 2010;20:929–36.

16. Lee WJ, Chong K, Ser KH, et al. C-peptide predicts the remission of type 2 diabetes after bariatric surgery. Obes Surg. 2012;22:293–8.

17. Livhits M, Mercado C, Yermilov I, et al. Preoperative predictors of weight loss following bariatric surgery: systematic review. Obes Surg. 2012;22:70–89.

18. Lomanto D, Lee WJ, Goel R, et al. Bariatric surgery in Asia in the last 5 years (2005–2009). Obes Surg. 2012;22:502–6.

19. Nguyen NT, Masoomi H, Laugenour K, et al. Predictive factors of mortality in bariatric surgery: data from the nationwide inpatient sample. Surgery. 2011;150:347–51.

20. O'Keeffe T, Patterson EJ. Evidence supporting routine polysomnography before bariatric surgery. Obes Surg. 2004;14:23–6.

21. Pontiroli AE, Morabito A. Long-term prevention of mortality in morbid obesity through bariatric surgery. A systematic review and meta-analysis of trials performed with gastric banding and gastric bypass. Ann Surg. 2011;253:484–7.

22. Pratt JS, Lenders CM, Dionne EA, et al. Best practice updates for pediatric/adolescent weight loss surgery. Obesity (Silver Spring). 2009;17:901–10.

23. Rocha IE, Victor EG, Braga MC, et al. Echocardiography evaluation for asymptomatic patients with severe obesity. Arq Bras Cardiol. 2007;88:52–8.

24. SAGES Guidelines Committee. SAGES guideline for clinical application of laparoscopic bariatric surgery. Surg Endosc. 2008;22:2281–300.

25. Sakcak I, Avsar FM, Cosgun E, et al. Management of concomitant cholelithiasis in gastric banding for morbid obesity. Eur J Gastroenterol Hepatol. 2011;23:766–9.

26. Sauerland S, Angrisani L, Belachew M, et al. Obesity surgery. Evidence-based guidelines of the European Association for Endoscopic Surgery (EAES). Surg Endosc. 2005;19:200–21.

27. Spyropoulos C, Kehagias I, Panagiotopoulos S, et al. Revisional bariatric surgery: 13-year experience from a tertiary institution. Arch Surg. 2010;145:173–7.

28. Tariq N, Chand B. Presurgical evaluation and postoperative care for the bariatric patient. Gastrointest Endosc Clin N Am. 2011;21:229–40.

29. Tarnoff M, Kim J, Shikora S. Patient selection, preoperative assessment, and preparation. In: Schauer PR, Schirmer BD, Brethauer SA, editors. Minimally invasive bariatric surgery. 1st ed. New York: Springer Science; 2007.

30. Umeura N, Okamoto S, Yamamoto S, et al. *Helicobacter pylori* infection and the development of gastric cancer. N Engl J Med. 2001;345:784–9.

31. Vaziri K, Bhanot P, Hungness ES, et al. Retrievable inferior vena cava filters in high-risk patients undergoing bariatric surgery. Surg Endosc. 2009;23:2203–7.

Why Are Bariatric Surgeries Risky?

Susumu Inamine

3.1 Introduction

Bariatric surgery is the only effective treatment that has been demonstrated to have long-lasting effects for morbidly obese individuals. Due to the increase in the obese population worldwide, the surgical treatment for morbid obesity has been increasing rapidly. It has been reported that more than 340,000 bariatric and metabolic surgeries were performed around the world in 2011. The number of procedures is expected to increase steadily in the future.

The perioperative morbidities and mortality rates of bariatric surgery for morbid obesity have been reported to be favorable compared to those of other major surgical procedures. Weight loss surgeries consist of relatively simple procedures for general surgeons who are familiar with modifying the digestive tract. However, such surgeries are far from easy. Because of the peculiar physical and functional characteristics of the morbidly obese individual, it has been said that bariatric surgery is one of the most challenging operations (Fig. 3.1). In addition, morbidly obese patients often have multiple comorbidities that can increase the risk of morbidity and mortality during the perioperative period. It is also known that morbidly obese patients have an increased risk of specific difficulties related to anesthesia.

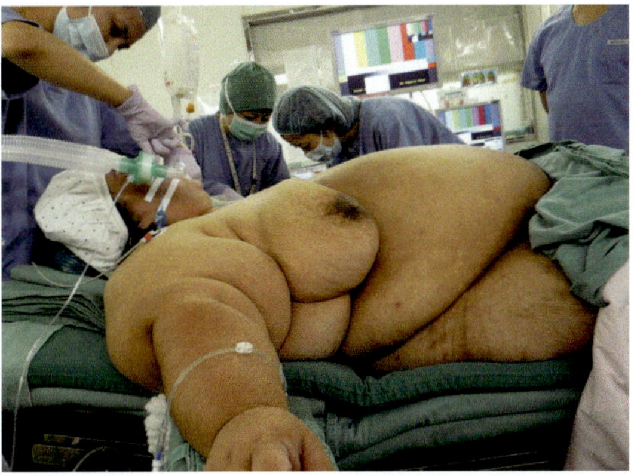

Fig. 3.1 Morbidly obese patient (BMI71)

In addition, since surgical treatment is occasionally related to postoperative complications, it is important to deal with these as well. However, in morbidly obese individuals, treating these postoperative complications is not easy as in non-obese patients because of their physical and functional differences. In this chapter, the reasons why bariatric procedures are risky will be described.

3.2 Comorbidities in Patients with Morbid Obesity

Morbid obesity is a potentially deadly situation that is a harbinger of multiple diseases and disorders, affecting every organ and system of the human body (Table 3.1). Several of these problems are described in detail below.

S. Inamine, MD
Department of Endoscopic Surgery, Nakagami
General Hospital, Okinawa, Japan
e-mail: soohs@mac.com

S.H. Choi, K. Kasama (eds.), *Bariatric and Metabolic Surgery*,
DOI 10.1007/978-3-642-35591-2_3, © Springer-Verlag Berlin Heidelberg 2014

Table 3.1 Comorbid medical conditions associated with morbid obesity

Cardiovascular
Hypertension
Congestive heart failure
Prolonged QT
Venous stasis
Deep venous thrombosis
Pulmonary hypertension
Pulmonary
Obstructive sleep apnea
Asthma
Hypoventilation syndrome
Metabolic
Type II diabetes
Hyperlipidemia
Hypercholesterolemia
Gastrointestinal
Gastroesophageal reflux
Choleolithiasis
Non-alcoholic steatotic hepatitis (NASH)
Psychiatric
Depression

3.2.1 Cardiovascular Problems

Cardiovascular dysfunction is commonly seen in morbidly obese patients and is manifested as hypertension and coronary artery disease. Heart failure may be the consequence of left or right ventricular hypertrophy secondary to hypertension. In addition, prolonged QT and sudden death syndrome occur more commonly in patients who are morbidly obese than in those who are not. Other cardiovascular problems include arrhythmia, ischemic stroke, and deep vein thrombosis with or without pulmonary embolus.

3.2.2 Respiratory Insufficiency

Respiratory insufficiency in patients with morbid obesity is associated with obstructive sleep apnea syndrome and obesity-hypoventilation syndrome. In these patients, abnormalities in respiratory function tests and arterial blood gas analyses can be seen. These abnormalities may cause systemic hypertension, pulmonary hypertension and

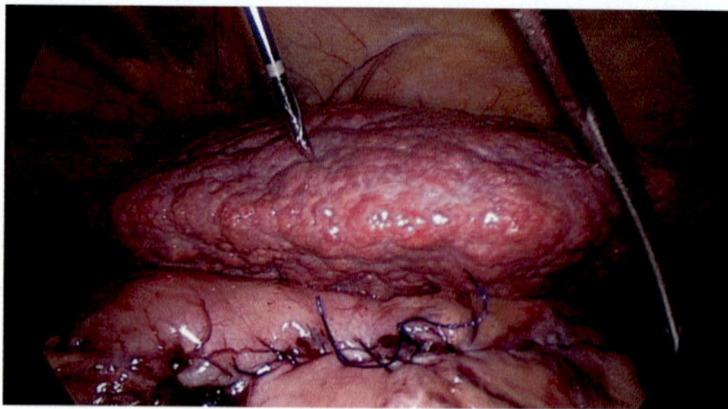

Fig. 3.2 Liver cirrhosis secondary to NASH in morbidly obese patient

cor pulmonale. In addition, obstructive sleep apnea may cause acute respiratory arrest and other life-threatening events.

3.2.3 Metabolic Complications

The relationship between central obesity and the constellation of health problems such as hypertension, hyperglycemia, and hyperlipidemia, known as "metabolic syndrome," is well established. It is thought that the increase of visceral fat causes insulin resistance, which subsequently causes hyperglycemia and hyperinsulinemia and finally leads to the development of type 2 diabetes mellitus. It has also been established that such conditions are responsible for nonalcoholic steatohepatitis (NASH), which can progress to liver cirrhosis (Fig. 3.2). Bariatric surgeons should also pay attention to the presence of renal dysfunction or failure secondary to type 2 diabetes. In the perioperative period, poor glycemic control can cause postoperative mortality secondary to comorbidities such as leakage at the site of gastrointestinal anastomosis, delayed wound healing, and surgical site infection. Other possible metabolic complications include hypertension, hyperlipidemia, and the formation of gall stones.

3.2.4 Other Comorbid Conditions

In patients who are morbidly obese, chronic lower limb venous stasis and hypercoagulability are often observed. These conditions may increase the risk of deep venous thrombosis and pulmonary embolus, which accounts for nearly half of the perioperative mortality due to bariatric surgery.

3.3 Issues Related to Anesthesia and Analgesia

In bariatric surgery patients, there are many problems related to anesthesia and analgesia. For example, the endotracheal intubation of these patients may be difficult even for experienced anesthesiologists. Changes in the structure of the oropharyngeal anatomy and reduced neck mobility make it difficult to control the airway for mask ventilation (Fig. 3.3). Moreover, narrowing of the pharyngeal space due to increased adipose tissue can make it difficult to obtain a good laryngoscopic view for endotracheal intubation. Oxygenation and ventilation are also compromised by the reduced compliance of the chest wall due to the significant increase of body fat. It is also known that morbidly obese patients are frequently hypoxic, with a marked decrease in their functional residual capacity (FRC) and expiratory reserve volume due to elevation of the diaphragm, especially in the supine position. The pharmacodynamics and pharmacokinetics of drugs used for anesthesia are different between severely obese patients and normal populations. In addition, the access to the arteries and central veins for monitoring and drug administration is often difficult because of the thick subcutaneous fat.

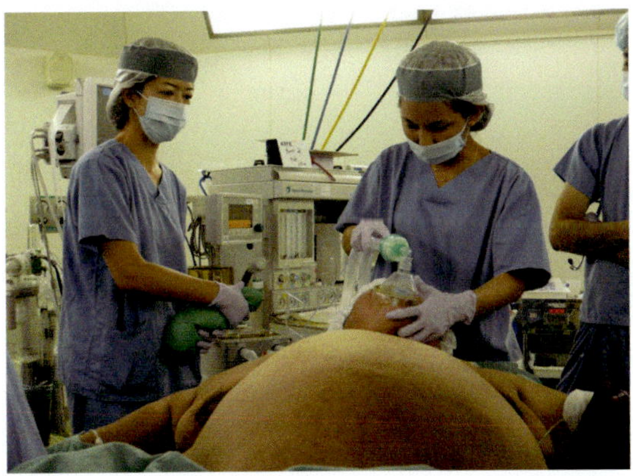

Fig. 3.3 Mask ventilation in super obese patient

3.4 Issues Related to Surgical Procedures

It may seem that the bariatric procedure itself should be easy for general surgeons who are familiar with laparoscopic gastrointestinal surgeries. Indeed, it could be said that bariatric procedures are simple. However, because of the physical features of the obese patients and characteristics of the surgery itself, the bariatric surgeries are relatively difficult (Table 3.2). Currently, the majority of weight loss surgery is done laparoscopically. However, the fairly thick abdominal wall of the patients can lead to difficulties with the access port, especially the first access (Fig. 3.4). The insertion of the first access port may lead to serious consequences, such as erroneous puncture of mesenteric blood vessels, the digestive tract, or retroperitoneal structures. In addition, the thickened abdominal wall can handcuff the access ports, and as a result, manipulation of the surgical instruments and telescope are limited (Fig. 3.5). Also, the markedly enlarged left lobe of the liver associated with obesity makes it difficult to ensure the appropriate working space and critical view around the angle of His, which is one of the most important points of the bariatric procedures (Fig. 3.6).

Moreover, the large amount of visceral fat and very thick omentum can give strong resistance to maneuvering the laparoscopic surgical instruments and narrows the working space for surgery in the abdominal cavity. Increasing the pressure of the pneumoperitoneum in order to ensure the abdominal space can lead to a risk of thrombosis and pulmonary complications. In addition, surgeons

Table 3.2 Surgical problems in bariatric surgery

Thick abdominal wall
Difficulty of trocar insertion especially first access
Limitation of laparoscopic surgical instruments maneuver
Enlarged left lobe of liver
Difficult to ensure the working space and critical view around the angle of His
Large amount of visceral fat
Narrow working space
Need relatively high pressure pneumoperitoneum

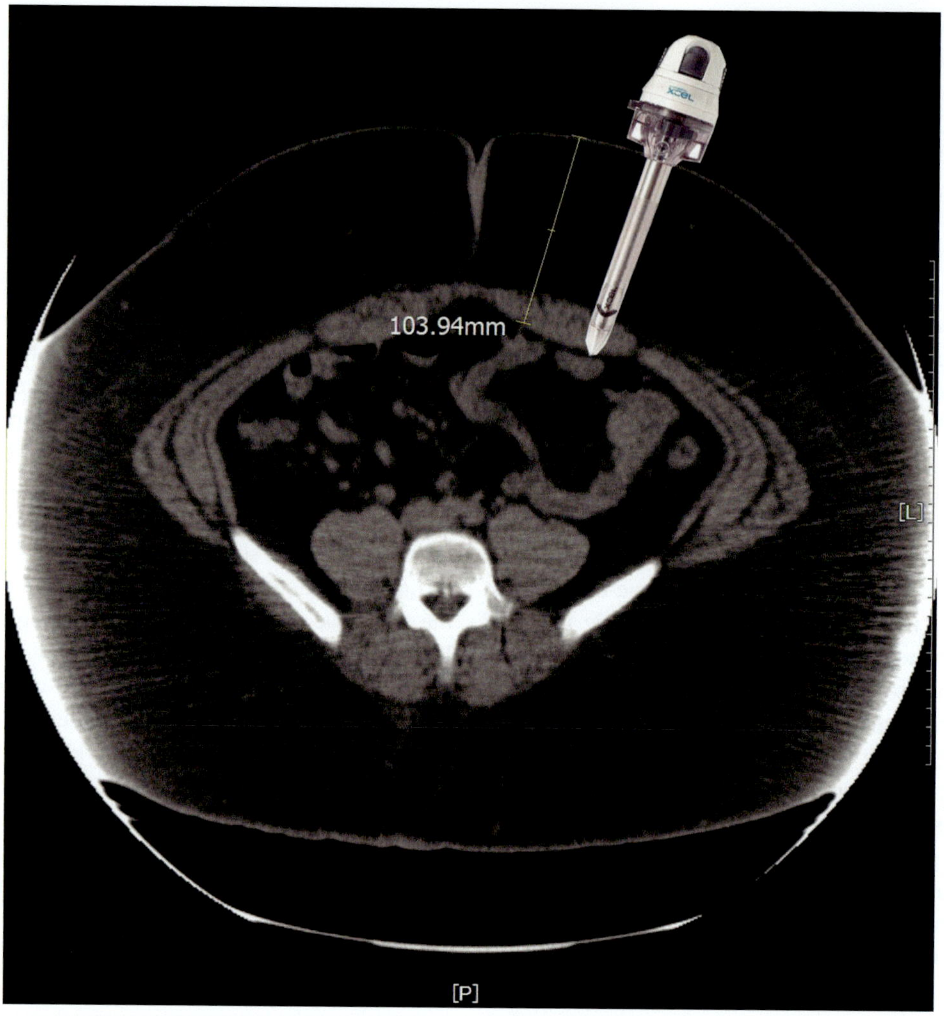

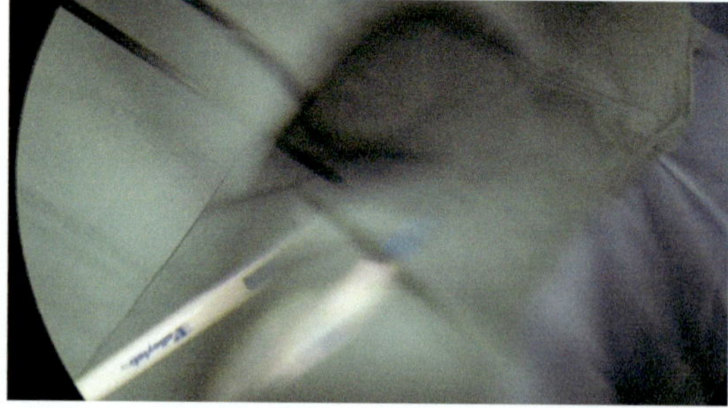

Fig. 3.4 CT shows fairly tick abdominal wall in super obese patient. Trocar is same scale

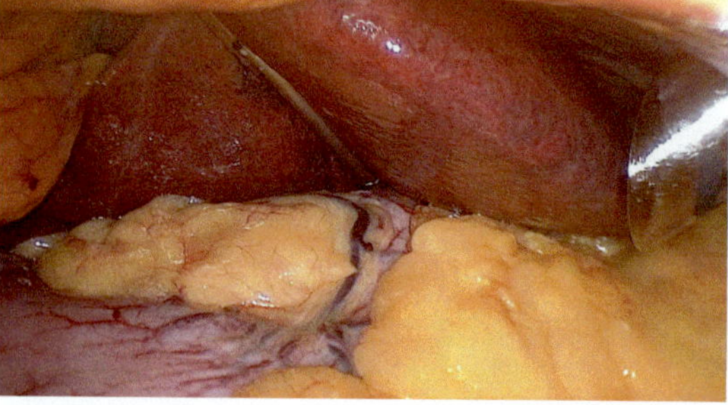

Fig. 3.5 Laparoscopic view of broken telescope due to tick abdominal wall resistance

Fig. 3.6 Markedly enlarged left lobe of the liver and large amount of visceral fat associated with obesity

should also keep in mind that the surgery for morbid obesity is not made easier by a conversion to an open procedure. Weight loss surgeries converted to laparotomy may amplify the deterioration of the deep site vision and the difficulty of the surgical procedure. For these reasons, if possible, the laparoscopic surgeon should complete all procedures laparoscopically. In addition, in order to obtain a sufficient weight loss effect, the size and shape of the gastric sleeve, gastric pouch, and stoma size need to be accurately adjusted laparoscopically. This is another factor that reduces the safety margin of bariatric surgery.

3.5   Difficulty Dealing with Postoperative Complications

As with other surgical procedures, it is not possible to completely eliminate the incidence of postoperative morbidities in bariatric surgery. Especially in bariatric patients, it is difficult to both deal with the perioperative comorbidities and also to obtain an early precise diagnosis. The diagnosis and treatment of postoperative complications in morbidly obese patients are described elsewhere.

Conclusions

Weight loss surgery for morbidly obese patients has been proven to be safe and effective. However, most patients who are candidates for bariatric surgery have some physical and functional characteristics that may lead to serious life-threatening perioperative morbidities. In order to provide effective and safe surgeries for these patients, bariatric surgeons must put a great deal of effort into improving the surgical procedures. In addition, it is also necessary to understand the characteristics of the bariatric patients. After a thorough risk assessment for each patient, the bariatric staff should endeavor to reduce the risk as much as possible prior to surgery.

Bibliography

1. Sjostrom L. Review of the key results from the Swedish Obese Subjects (SOS) trial – a prospective controlled intervention study of bariatric surgery. J Intern Med. 2013;273(3):219–34.
2. Buchwald H, Oien DM. Metabolic/bariatric surgery worldwide 2011. Obes Surg. 2013;23(4):427.
3. Buchwald H, Avidor Y, et al. Bariatric surgery: a systemic review and analysis. JAMA. 2004;292(14):1724.
4. Maggard MA, Shugamann LR, et al. Meta-analysis: surgical treatment of obesity. Ann Intern Med. 2005; 142(7):547.
5. Buchwald H, Esok R. Trends in mortality in bariatric surgery: a systematic review and meta-analysis. Surgery. 2007;142(4):621.
6. Lancaster RH, Hutter MM. Bands and bypass: 30-day morbidity and mortality of bariatric surgical procedures assessment by prospective, multi-center, risk-adjusted ACS-NSQIP data. Surg Endosc. 2008;22(12):2554.
7. Stein PD, Matta F. Pulmonary embolism and deep venous thrombosis following bariatric surgery. Obes Surg. 2013;23(5):663.
8. Higa KD, Boone KB, Ho T. Complications of the laparoscopic Roux-en-Y gastric bypass: 1,040 patients – what have we learned? Obes Surg. 2000;10:509.
9. Morino M, Toppino M, Forestieri P, et al. Mortality after bariatric surgery: analysis of 13,871 morbidly obese patients from a national registry. Ann Surg. 2007;246:1002.
10. Konrad FM, et al. Anesthesia and bariatric surgery. Anaesthetist. 2011;60(7):607–16.

Yosuke Seki

4.1 NIH Criteria

The National Institutes of Health (NIH) criteria for patient selection for gastrointestinal surgery for severe obesity were developed in 1991 at a consensus conference involving expert surgeons, gastroenterologists, endocrinologists, psychiatrists, nutritionists and other health-care professionals, as well as the public [1]. After weighing the evidence, the panel made the following recommendations:

1. Patients seeking therapy for severe obesity for the first time should be considered for treatment in a nonsurgical program with integrated components of a dietary regimen, appropriate exercise, and behavioral modification and support.
2. Gastric restrictive or bypass procedures could be considered for well-informed and motivated patients with acceptable operative risks.
3. Patients who are candidates for surgical procedures should be selected carefully after evaluation by a multidisciplinary team with medical, surgical, psychiatric, and nutritional expertise.
4. The operation should be performed by a surgeon substantially experienced with the appropriate procedures and working in a clini-

cal setting with adequate support for all aspects of management and assessment.
5. Lifelong medical surveillance after surgical therapy is necessary to monitor for complications and lifestyle adjustments.

In short, the patient selection criteria recommendations were that surgery is an option for well-informed and motivated patients who have "clinically severe obesity," indicated by a body mass index (BMI) 40 kg/m², or a BMI 35 kg/m², and serious comorbid conditions.

Although these criteria were established more than 20 years ago, they continue to be the most quoted and used. Many surgical societies, health-care service providers, and third-party payers around the world have adopted very similar, or at times more restrictive, eligibility criteria for bariatric surgery.

4.2 ASMBS Statements/ Guidelines in Class I Obesity

Since the NIH consensus conference of 1991, new procedures have been introduced, the laparoscopic approach has largely replaced open surgery, and higher levels of scientific evidence are available regarding the health hazards of obesity and the risks and benefits of bariatric surgery. In response to this, the ASMBS (American Society for Metabolic and Bariatric Surgery) Clinical Issues Committee has most recently issued the following position statements regarding bariatric surgery in Class I obesity (BMI 30–35 kg/m²)

Y. Seki, MD
Head of Obesity and Diabetes Research Unit,
Weight Loss and Metabolic Surgery Center,
Yotsuya Medical Cube, Tokyo, Japan
e-mail: seki@mcube.jp

S.H. Choi, K. Kasama (eds.), *Bariatric and Metabolic Surgery*,
DOI 10.1007/978-3-642-35591-2_4, © Springer-Verlag Berlin Heidelberg 2014

based on current knowledge, expert opinion, and published peer-reviewed scientific evidence [2]:

1. Class I obesity is a well-defined disease that causes or exacerbates multiple other diseases, decreases lifespan, and decreases quality of life. A patient with Class I obesity should be recognized as deserving treatment for this disease.
2. Current options of nonsurgical treatment for Class I obesity are not generally effective in achieving substantial and durable weight reduction.
3. For patients with BMI 30–35 kg/m^2 who do not achieve substantial and durable weight and comorbidity improvement with nonsurgical methods, bariatric surgery should be an available option for suitable individuals. The existing cutoff of BMI, which excludes those with Class I obesity, was established arbitrarily nearly 20 years ago. There is no current justification on grounds of evidence of clinical effectiveness, cost-effectiveness, ethics, or equity that this group should be excluded from life-saving treatment.
4. Gastric banding, sleeve gastrectomy, and gastric bypass have been shown in randomized controlled trials to be well-tolerated and effective treatment for patients with BMI 30–35 kg/m^2 in the short and medium term.

4.3 Contraindication to Bariatric Surgery

There are no absolute contraindications to bariatric surgery. Relative contraindications to surgery may include severe heart failure, unstable coronary artery disease, end-stage lung disease, active cancer diagnosis/treatment, cirrhosis with portal hypertension, uncontrolled drug or alcohol dependency, and severely impaired intellectual capacity. Crohn's disease may be a relative contraindication to Roux-en-Y gastric bypass (RYGB) and biliopancreatic diversion (BPD) and is listed by the manufacturer as a contraindication to adjustable gastric banding (AGB).

4.3.1 Age

Traditionally, surgeons offered bariatric surgery to patients aged 18–60 years. However, in the current era of refined anesthesiology, effective critical care, and high-quality surgical outcomes, age restrictions are less rigidly employed. Laparoscopic bariatric surgery has been performed in patients older than 55–60 years [3–5], but with less weight loss, longer length of hospitalization, higher morbidity and mortality, and less complete resolution of comorbidities compared with younger patients. Still, the reduction in comorbidities supports use of laparoscopic RYGB or laparoscopic AGB in well-selected older patients [6–13].

On the other hand, bariatric surgery for morbidly obese children and adolescents was not advised because of insufficient data at the NIH consensus conference in 1991. However, with pediatric obesity increasing in prevalence and severity, interest in adolescent bariatric surgery is growing [14]. RYGB is well tolerated and produces excellent weight loss in patients younger than 18 years with a 10-year follow-up [15–21]. Advocates believe weight reduction at an early age will prevent or minimize emotional and physical consequences of obesity [22]. Well-designed prospective studies are just emerging to better define the place for adolescent bariatric surgery [23].

4.3.2 Ethnicity

BMI is used as a surrogate for adiposity and as a marker for risk associated with increasing body weight. However, there are major ethnic differences in both the degree of adiposity and risk of obesity-related diseases. That is, Asian populations have a higher percentage of body fat for a given weight and are predisposed to abdominal adiposity. Accumulation of visceral fat occurs at lower BMIs, increasing the risks of hypertension, dyslipidemia, diabetes, and metabolic syndrome. The prevalence of Type II diabetes in Asia is similar to that of Western countries, although the average BMI in Asia is lower. Recently, the World Health Organization (WHO) consultation has recommended that for those with Asian ethnicity, public health BMI action points may be reduced by 2.0–2.5 kg/m^2 to 23.0, 27.5, 32.5, and 37.5 kg/m^2 [24]. Recognizing the increased adiposity and comorbidity risk, the WHO and International Obesity Task Force (IOTF) have also recognized an increased risk of Type II diabetes at lower BMI levels in Asian populations [25], and the International Diabetes Federation (IDF) has used ethnic-specific waist circumferences for men and women when defining the metabolic syndrome [26].

Ethnic differences in adiposity and disease risk should be considered in determining indications for bariatric surgery. In 2005, the Asia-Pacific Bariatric Surgery Group (APBSG) consensus meeting was held and recommended bariatric surgery in Asian patients with BMI >37 or >32 kg/m^2 with diabetes or two other obesity-related comorbidities [27]. Subsequently, in 2011, International Federation for the Surgery of Obesity and Metabolic Disorders, Asia-Pacific Chapter (IFSO-APC) consensus statements as a renewed indication for Asian patients were established as follows [28]:

1. Bariatric surgery should be considered for the treatment of obesity for acceptable Asian candidates with BMI $\geq$35 kg/m^2 with or without comorbidities.
2. Bariatric/GI metabolic surgery should be considered for the treatment of Type II diabetes or metabolic syndrome for patients who are inadequately controlled by lifestyle alternations and medical treatment for acceptable Asian candidates with BMI $\geq$30 kg/m^2.
3. The surgical approach may be considered as a non-primary alternative to treat inadequately controlled Type II diabetes, or metabolic syndrome, for suitable Asian candidates with BMI $\geq$27.5 kg/m^2.

References

1. Gastrointestinal surgery for severe obesity: National Institute of Health Consensus Development Conference statement. Am J Clin Nutr. 1992;55:615S–19S.
2. ASMBS Clinical Issues Committee. Bariatric surgery in class I obesity (body mass index 30–35 kg/m2). Surg Obes Relat Dis. 2013;9:e1–10.
3. Hazzan D, Chin EH, Steinhagen E, et al. Laparoscopic bariatric surgery can be safe for treatment of morbid obesity in patients older than 60 years. Surg Obes Relat Dis. 2006;2(6):613–6.
4. Papasavas PK, Gagne DJ, Kelly J, et al. Laparoscopic Roux-en-Y gastric bypass is a safe and effective operation for the treatment of morbid obesity in patients older than 55 years. Obes Surg. 2004;14(8):1056–61.
5. Frutos MD, Luján J, Hernández Q, et al. Results of laparoscopic gastric bypass in patients > or =55 years old. Obes Surg. 2006;16(4):461–4.
6. St Peter SD, Craft RO, Tided JL, et al. Impact of advanced age on weight loss and health benefits after laparoscopic gastric bypass. Arch Surg. 2005;140(2):165–8.
7. Varela JE, Wilson SE, Nguyen NT. Outcomes of bariatric surgery in the elderly. Am Surg. 2006;72(10):865–9.
8. Dunkle-Blatter SE, St Jean MR, Whitehead C, et al. Outcomes among elderly bariatric patients at a high-volume center. Surg Obes Relat Dis. 2007;3(2):163–9.
9. Flum DR, Salem L, Elrod JA, et al. Early mortality among Medicare beneficiaries undergoing bariatric surgical procedures. JAMA. 2005;294(15):1903–8.
10. Sosa JL, Pombo H, Pallavicini H, et al. Laparoscopic gastric bypass beyond age 60. Obes Surg. 2004;14(10):1398–401.
11. Sugerman HJ, DeMaria EJ, Kellum JM, et al. Effects of bariatric surgery in older patients. Ann Surg. 2004;240(2):243–7.
12. Taylor CJ, Layani L. Laparoscopic adjustable gastric banding in patients C60 years old: is it worthwhile? Obes Surg. 2006;16(12):1579–83.
13. Quebbemann B, Engstrom D, Siegfried T. Bariatric surgery in patients older than 65 years is safe and effective. Surg Obes Relat Dis. 2005;1(4):389–92.
14. Allen SR, Lawson L, Garcia V, et al. Attitudes of bariatric surgeons concerning adolescent bariatric surgery. Obes Surg. 2005;15:1192–5.
15. Sanford A, Glascock JM, Eid GM, et al. Laparoscopic Roux-en-Y gastric bypass in morbidly obese adolescents. J Pediatr Surg. 2003;38:430–3.
16. Inge TH, Garcia VF, Daniels SR, et al. A multidisciplinary approach to the adolescent bariatric surgical patient. J Pediatr Surg. 2004;39:442–7.
17. Strauss RS, Bradley LJ, Brolin RE. Gastric bypass surgery in adolescents with morbid obesity. J Pediatr. 2001;138:499–504.
18. Breaux CW. Obesity surgery in children. Obes Surg. 1995;5:279–84.
19. Rand CS, Macgregor AM. Adolescents having obesity surgery: a 6 year follow-up. South Med J. 1994;87:1208–13.
20. Sugerman HJ, Sugerman EL, Demaria EJ. Bariatric surgery for severely obese adolescents. J Gastrointest Surg. 2003;7:102–8.

21. Barnett SJ, Stanley S, Hanlon M, et al. Long-term follow-up and the role of surgery in adolescents with morbid obesity. Surg Obes Relat Dis. 2005;1:394–8.
22. Capella JF, Capella RF. Bariatric surgery in adolescence. Is this the best age to operate? Obes Surg. 2003;13:826–32.
23. Inge TH, Xanthakos SA, Zeller MH. Bariatric surgery for pediatric extreme obesity: now or later? Int J Obes. 2007;31:1–14.
24. WHO Expert Consultation. Appropriate body-mass index for Asian populations and its implications for policy and intervention strategies. Lancet. 2004;363(9403):157–63.
25. Misra A, Wasir JS, Vikram NK. Waist circumference criteria for the diagnosis of abdominal obesity are not applicable uniformly to all populations and ethnic groups. Nutrition. 2005;21(9):969–76.
26. Ford ES. Prevalence of the metabolic syndrome defined by the International Diabetes Federation among adults in the U.S. Diabetes Care. 2005;28(11):2745–9.
27. Lee WJ, Wang W. Bariatric surgery: Asia-Pacific perspective. Obes Surg. 2005;15:751–7.
28. Kasama K, Lee WJ, Seki Y, et al. IFSO-APC consensus statements 2011. Obes Surg. 2012;22(5):677–84.

Part II

Surgical Techniques and Tips

Takeshi Naitoh

5.1 Equipment for Laparoscopic Bariatric Surgery

5.1.1 Laparoscopic Equipment

Bariatric surgeries are mostly performed by the laparoscopic procedures, at the present. Laparoscopic surgery system is including a laparoscopic camera system, a light source, an insufflator, and display monitors. The development of today's technology has resulted in a variety of innovations in the field of surgical equipment.

5.1.1.1 Camera System and Display Monitor

The camera system for the laparoscopic surgery has dramatically changed in recent years. The high-definition camera system whose resolution is 1920×1080 dpi has enabled the presentation of detailed images, and it leads to perform the precise operation.

The endoscope for the bariatric surgery should be able to present the perspective view, such as $30°$ telescope or flexible endoscope. A 5-mm telescope is not suitable for bariatric surgeries because the thickened abdominal wall would sometimes disturb the motion of the telescope, and it would break when panning or tilting a scope. The display monitor is also important. It

T. Naitoh, MD, FACS
Department of Surgery, Tohoku University Hospital, Sendai, Japan
e-mail: naitot@surg1.med.tohoku.ac.jp

should be able to display the high-definition images without losing image quality.

5.1.1.2 Insufflator
The laparoscopic insufflator is also required. The max gas flow speed should be at least 20 L/min, to prevent the collapse of the surgical space when using suction.

5.1.1.3 Light Source
The light source and light guide cable are not different from the regular laparoscopic equipment. The xenon light source is commonly used.

5.1.2 Laparoscopic Instrument

5.1.2.1 Trocar
A trocar used for bariatric surgeries is not basically different from the regular one. However, since the abdominal wall of the patient is sometimes more than 10 cm in thickness, the longer trocar is required (Fig. 5.1). Regarding a diameter of the trocar, we recommend the 12-mm one. The 5-mm trocar could be used for tissue dissection or liver retraction, but a laparoscopic linear stapler can be inserted only through the trocar in which the diameter is more than 12 mm, and a 26-mm half-circle suture needle which is typically used for bariatric surgery cannot be inserted through the 5-mm trocar. Besides, if performing the sleeve gastrectomy, a one 15-mm trocar is indispensable for extracting the resected stomach. Furthermore, for the first trocar entry, the

S.H. Choi, K. Kasama (eds.), *Bariatric and Metabolic Surgery*,
DOI 10.1007/978-3-642-35591-2_5, © Springer-Verlag Berlin Heidelberg 2014

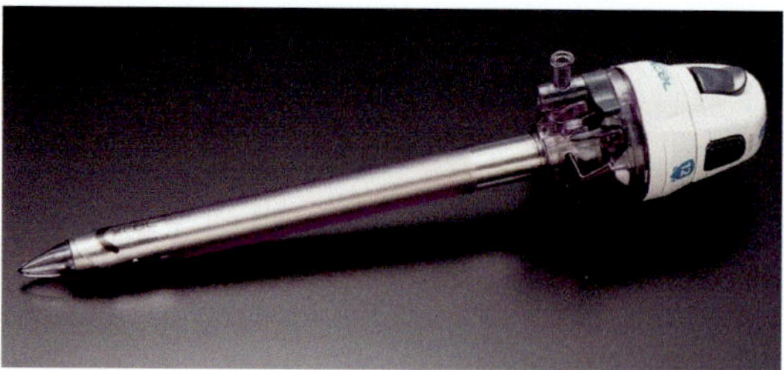

Fig. 5.1 A trocar used for bariatric surgeries is not basically different from the regular one. However, since the abdominal wall of the patient is sometimes more than 10 cm in thickness, the longer trocar is required

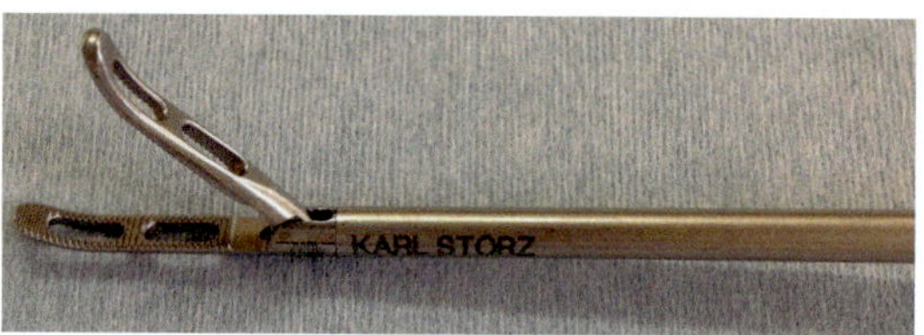

Fig. 5.2 The laparoscopic bowel grasper, fenestrated atraumatic long-jaw forceps

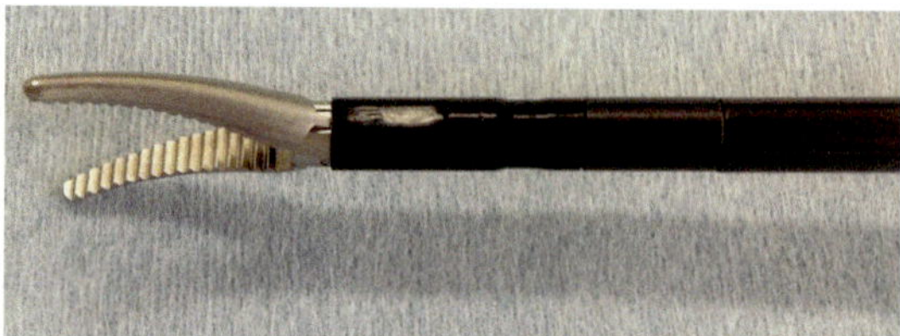

Fig. 5.3 The Maryland-type dissecting forceps

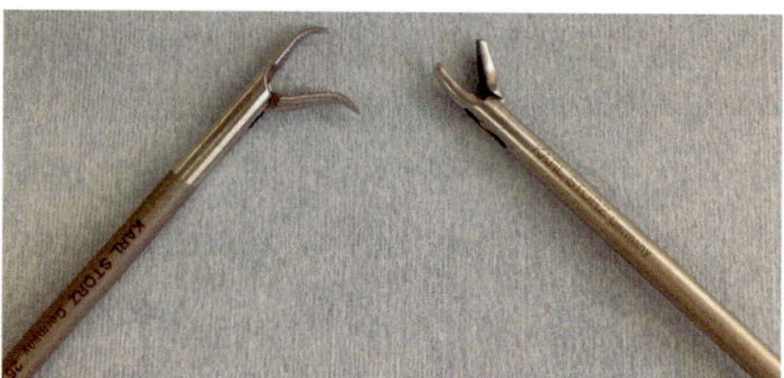

Fig. 5.4 Needle holder

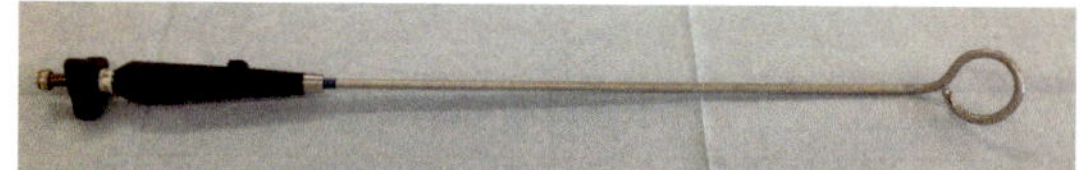

Fig. 5.5 Snake-type retractor

optical access trocar is strongly recommended, since the blind insertion of a Veress needle or the Hasson method is extremely difficult.

5.1.2.2 Grasper

The laparoscopic bowel grasper is mainly used for bariatric surgeries. A couple of bowel graspers should be prepared. There are some variations of bowel grasper offered from each company but basically the fenestrated atraumatic long-jaw forceps (Fig. 5.2). A Debakey-type forceps is often used for suturing. They are all 5-mm instruments in diameter.

A 10-mm claw forceps is required for extracting the resected stomach when performing the sleeve gastrectomy.

A ratchet handle for the grasper is not crucial but recommended.

5.1.2.3 Dissector

The Maryland-type dissecting forceps is commonly used. The right-angle dissector might be needed (Fig. 5.3).

5.1.2.4 Needle Holder

Bariatric surgeries require intracorporeal suturing and knot-tying technique in various situa-

tions. Therefore, a needle driver is essential (Fig. 5.4). There are many types of laparoscopic needle drivers commercially available. It depends on a surgeon's preference what kind of needle holder is chosen. However, it is important to select what is easy to handle.

5.1.2.5 Retractor

The retractor is mostly used for liver retraction. In morbid obesity patients, the liver is often fatty and swollen due to severe fatty liver or nonalcoholic steatohepatitis (NASH), and it results in poor visibility of surgical field. Therefore, a sturdy 5-mm fan-type or snake-type retractor is required (Fig. 5.5).

A gastric banding retractor sold by Karl Storz Inc. is useful for adjustable gastric banding, Roux-en-Y gastric bypass, and confirming the angle of His in case of sleeve gastrectomy (Fig. 5.6).

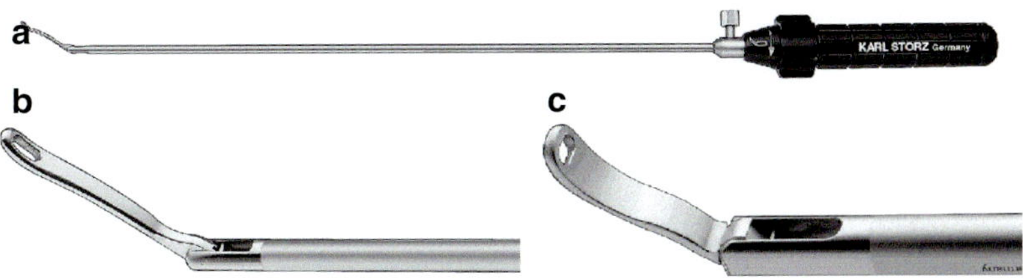

Fig. 5.6 Gastric banding retractor, Karl Storz, Inc. The tip of the retractor is blunt and it can be flexed (**a**). The product lineup consists of 5 mm (**b**) and 10 mm (**c**)

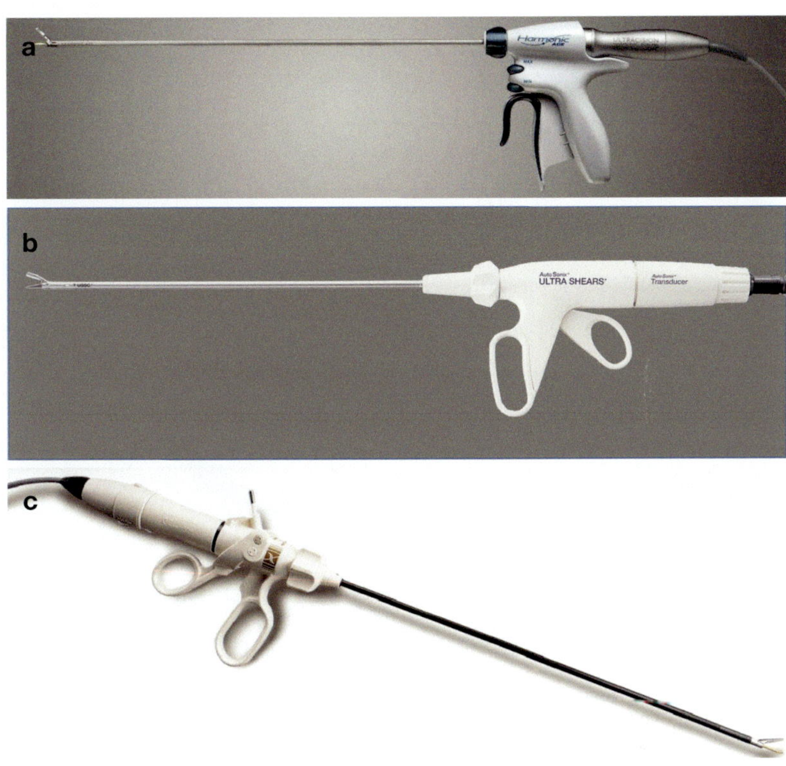

Fig. 5.7 Ultrasonic coagulating device. Harmonic Scalpel™, Ethicon Endo-Surgery Inc (**a**); AutoSonix™, Covidien Inc (**b**); and SonoSurg™, Olympus Co (**c**)

5.1.2.6 Energy Device

Energy devices utilized in bariatric surgeries are various. Electric cautery is essential as well as other laparoscopic surgeries to control minor oozing.

Laparoscopic ultrasonic coagulating shears (e.g., Harmonic Scalpel™, Ethicon Endo-Surgery Inc.; AutoSonix™, Covidien Inc.; and SonoSurg™, Olympus Co.) (Fig. 5.7) or bipolar-type sealing and cutting device (e.g., LigaSure™, Covidien Inc., or Enseal™, Ethicon Endo-Surgery Inc.) (Fig. 5.8) is required for dissection of vessels around the stomach or the intestinal mesentery to achieve secure hemostasis. The choice of device depends on the preference of the surgeon. Generally, ultrasonic devices can cut the tissue even at the tip of the device though hemostatic potential is limited. On the other hand, bipolar-type devices yield strong hemostasis compared to ultrasonic devices but are not suitable for precise short-pitch cutting. The length of device is also an important issue. Although the device with regular length would not allow to reach the deep area in case of bariatric surgery, there is an opposite problem that the longer device is not rigid enough.

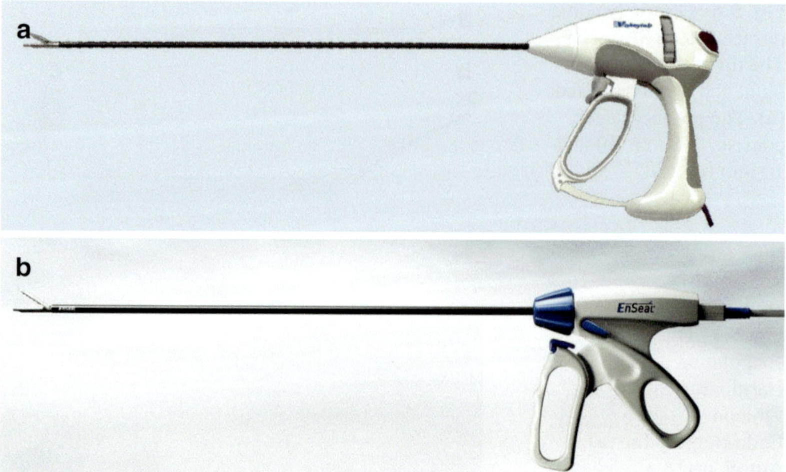

Fig. 5.8 Bipolar-type sealing and cutting system. LigaSure™, Covidien Inc (**a**); Enseal™, Ethicon Endo-Surgery Inc (**b**)

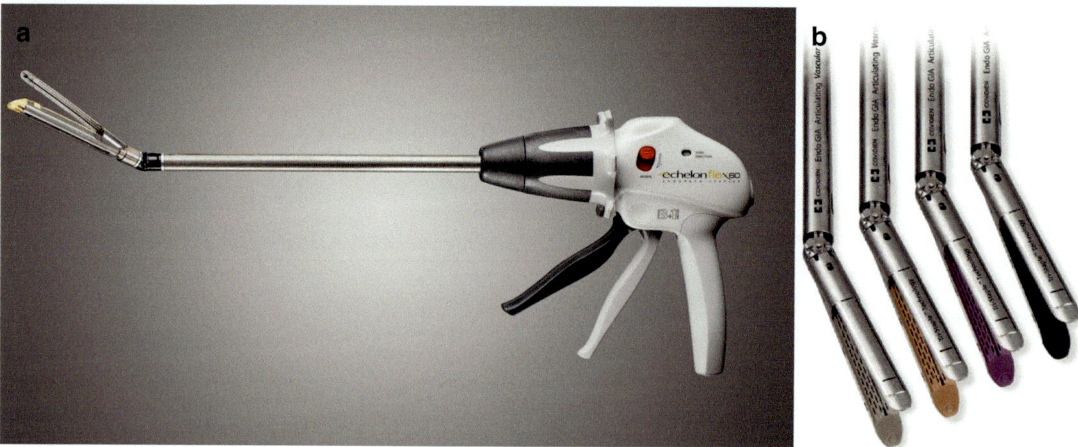

Fig. 5.9 Laparoscopic linear stapler. Echelon Flex™, Ethicon Endo-Surgery, Inc (**a**); Endo GIA™ Tri-Staple™ cartridge, Covidien, Inc (**b**)

5.1.2.7 Stapling Device

Laparoscopic stapling devices including the linear stapler (Fig. 5.9) and the circular stapler (Fig. 5.10) are essential devices in today's laparoscopic surgery. They provide better outcome in terms of reducing the operation time and securing the anastomosis. The laparoscopic linear stapler, in bariatric surgeries, is applied for various situations such as transection of the stomach or the small intestine, while the circular stapler is used only in limited situation.

When using the linear stapler, the proper staple size should be selected to accomplish the safe and secure transection. Thickness of the gastric wall is considered as thinner at the proximal side close to the esophagus and thicker around the antrum near the pylorus [4].

5.1.2.8 Suture

Reinforcement of the staple line after sleeve gastrectomy is performed by braded suture. A 2-0 or 3-0 braded suture, both absorbable and nonabsorbable, is commonly used. As it is usually performed by running fashion, a thread of approximately 20 cm in length is easy to handle. For the anastomosis of the digestive tract, a 3-0 absorbable braded suture is recommended. A 26-mm half-circle needle is preferred for both anastomosis and staple line reinforcement.

5.1.2.9 Gastric Bougie

Gastric bougie for sleeve gastrectomy or gastric bypass is inserted orally under general anesthesia before skin incision. This bougie is made of either

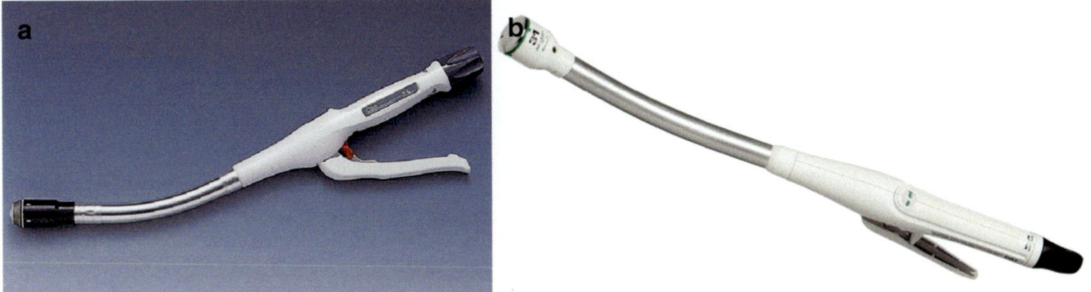

Fig. 5.10 Circular stapler. CDH stapler, Ethicon Endo-Surgery, Inc (**a**); EEA™ Stapler, Covidien, Inc (**b**)

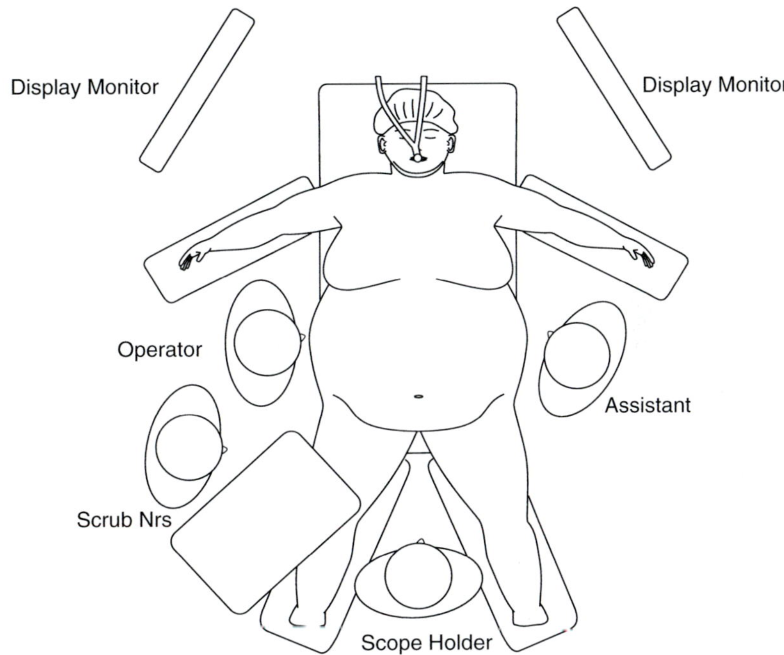

Fig. 5.11 The patient is placed in a supine with slightly leg split position. Usually, the operating surgeon stands at the right side of the patient, and the scope-holding surgeon stands between legs. Another surgeon stands at the left side of the patient, to assist the tissue retraction, and the scrub nurse stands at the right side of the patient next to the operating surgeon

plastic or rubber. Regarding the size of the bougie, it is still controversial whether the tighter bougie size results in a better weight loss effect. A 32–60-Fr. size bougie is generally applied [1, 8, 9, 11].

5.2 Position of the Patients and Operating Team

5.2.1 Patient Position

The patient is placed in a supine with slightly leg split position. Usually, the operating surgeon stands at the right side of the patient, and the scope-holding surgeon stands between legs. Another surgeon stands at left side of the patient, to assist the tis-sue retraction, and the scrub nurse stands at the right side of the patient next to the operating surgeon (Fig. 5.11). During the procedure, the patient is placed in a reverse Trendelenburg position [6]. Care should be taken to confirm that the patient stays at the proper position during surgery.

5.2.2 Preoperative Simulation

Preoperative simulation of patient setting is important. Since obese patients would easily complicate with skin trouble such as bed sore, it is strongly recommended to have an opportunity to check the discomfort while lying on the surgical bed, before surgery.

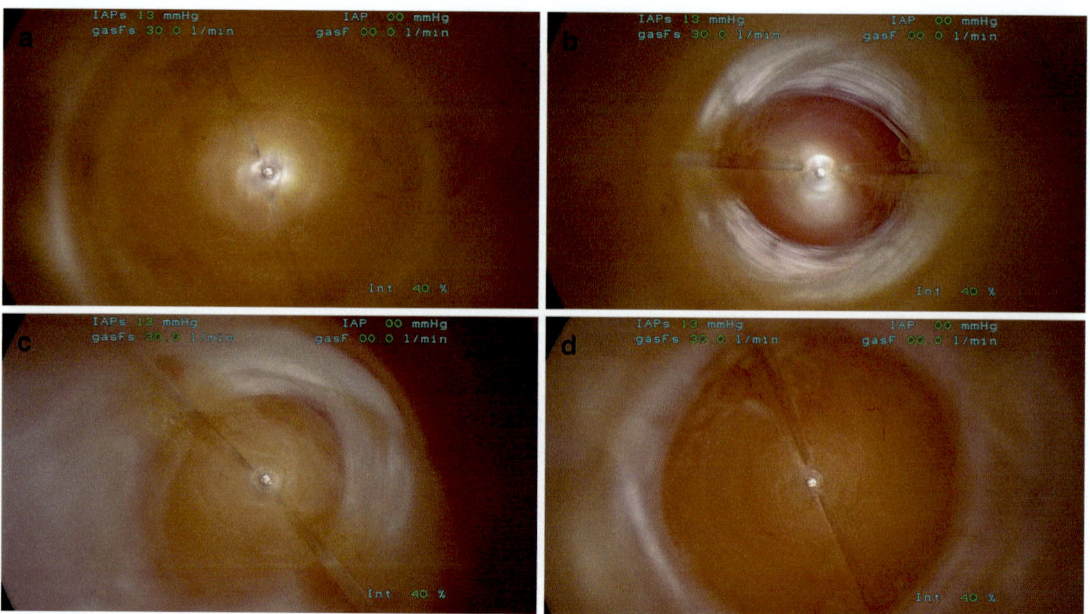

Fig. 5.12 The 0° telescope is inserted to the optical access trocar, then focusing a camera at the tip of the trocar. A small skin incision is created in the abdominal wall and the optical access trocar placed in the incision. The trocar is twisted so that the subcutaneous tissue is divided. Then the ventral fascia of the rectus sheath can be recognized as a white thick membrane (**a**). Once passing through the ventral fascia, the brown muscle tissue can be seen (**b**). Then, dividing the rectus muscle, preperitoneal adipose tissue will appear (**c**). By twisting and pushing the trocar gently, it will get into the abdominal cavity (**d**)

5.2.3 Operating Team

Operating team of bariatric surgery should be well trained and understand the procedure. Normally, the operating team includes 3 surgeons, 1 anesthesiologist, 1 scrub nurse, and 1 circumference nurse.

5.3 How to Make a Pneumoperitoneum in Morbid obese Patients

5.3.1 How to Create a Pneumoperitoneum

In bariatric surgeries, the first trocar insertion is a big issue. In the other laparoscopic procedure, a Hasson method is commonly applied to create the pneumoperitoneum and for the first trocar insertion. However, the thickness of the abdominal wall of morbidly obese patients sometimes becomes more than 10 cm, and it makes this technique difficult. The Veress needle technique is also difficult, because the abdominal cavity is very small even with the high-pressure pneumoperitoneum and the blind insertion of the first trocar is not able to guarantee the safety. Therefore, the optical access method is usually adopted to insert the first trocar [2, 3, 12]. Briefly, the 0° telescope is inserted into the optical access trocar, then focusing a camera at the tip of the trocar. A small skin incision is created in the abdominal wall and the optical access trocar placed in the incision. The trocar is twisted so that the subcutaneous tissue is divided. Then the ventral fascia of the rectus sheath can be recognized as a white thick membrane (Fig. 5.12a). Once passing through the ventral fascia, the brown muscle tissue can be seen (Fig. 5.12b). Then, dividing the rectus muscle, preperitoneal adipose tissue will appear (Fig. 5.12c). By twisting and pushing the trocar gently, it will get into the abdominal cavity (Fig. 5.12d). Removing the inner trocar, leaving the outer cannula, carbon dioxide gas can be insufflated and create the pneumoperitoneum. The surgeon should confirm that the cannula is properly placed into the abdominal cavity by viewing with the telescope.

5.3.2 Pressure

The intra-abdominal pressure should be kept around 10 mmHg during the surgery. When the surgeon had the difficulty in viewing with the regular pressure, the muscle relaxation should be checked at first. If the muscle relaxation is considered to be enough, then the intra-abdominal pressure might be elevated carefully. However, more than 15-mmHg pressure is not recommended because it enhances the risk of venous thrombosis, reduces venous blood flow, increases airway pressure, and impairs cardiac function [5, 7, 10].

References

1. Aurora AR, Khaitan L, Saber AA. Sleeve gastrectomy and the risk of leak: a systematic analysis of 4,888 patients. Surg Endosc. 2012;26(6):1509–15.
2. Berch BR, Torquati A, Lutfi RE, Richards WO. Experience with the optical access trocar for safe and rapid entry in the performance of laparoscopic gastric bypass. Surg Endosc. 2006;20(8):1238–41.
3. Bernante P, Foletto M, Toniato A. Creation of pneumoperitoneum using a bladed optical trocar in morbidly obese patients: technique and results. Obes Surg. 2008;18(8):1043–6.
4. Elariny H, González H, Wang B. Tissue thickness of human stomach measured on excised gastric specimens from obese patients. Surg Technol Int. 2005;14:119–24.
5. Guenoun T, Aka EJ, Journois D, Philippe H, Chevallier JM, Safran D. Effects of laparoscopic pneumoperitoneum and changes in position on arterial pulse pressure wave-form: comparison between morbidly obese and normal-weight patients. Obes Surg. 2006;16(8):1075–81.
6. Mulier JP, Dillemans B, Van Cauwenberge S. Impact of the patient's body position on the intraabdominal workspace during laparoscopic surgery. Surg Endosc. 2010;24(6):1398–402.
7. Nguyen NT, Wolfe BM. The physiologic effects of pneumoperitoneum in the morbidly obese. Ann Surg. 2005;241(2):219–26.
8. Parikh M, Gagner M, Heacock L, Strain G, Dakin G, Pomp A. Laparoscopic sleeve gastrectomy: does bougie size affect mean %EWL? Short-term outcomes. Surg Obes Relat Dis. 2008;4(4):528–33.
9. Parikh M, Issa R, McCrillis A, Saunders JK, Ude-Welcome A, Gagner M. Surgical strategies that may decrease leak after laparoscopic sleeve gastrectomy: a systematic review and meta-analysis of 9991 cases. Ann Surg. 2013;257(2):231–7.
10. Popescu WM, Bell R, Duffy AJ, Katz KH, Perrino Jr AC. A pilot study of patients with clinically severe obesity undergoing laparoscopic surgery: evidence for impaired cardiac performance. J Cardiothorac Vasc Anesth. 2011;25(6):943–9.
11. Rosenthal RJ, et al. International Sleeve Gastrectomy Expert Panel Consensus Statement: best practice guidelines based on experience of 12,000 cases. Surg Obes Relat Dis. 2012;8(1):8–19.
12. Sabeti N, Tarnoff M, Kim J, Shikora S. Primary midline peritoneal access with optical trocar is safe and effective in morbidly obese patients. Surg Obes Relat Dis. 2009;5(5):610–4.

Kazunori Kasama

6.1 Introduction

Since Wittgrove and Clark published their initial results on laparoscopic gastric bypass in 1993 [1], the procedure has seen an increase in acceptance around the world. Now, LRYGB (Fig. 6.1) is the most popular procedure in the field of bariatric surgery worldwide [2]. There is, however, no uniform way that LRYGB is performed. This is most noticeably reflected in the number of different ways in which gastrojejunostomy is performed as below:

1. Circular stapler anastomosis
2. Linear stapler anastomosis
3. Hand-suturing anastomosis

We prefer to perform using the hand-suturing anastomosis method, so the technique described in this chapter is based on LYRGB with hand-suturing gastrojejunostomy, but we would also like to describe all three anastomosis techniques.

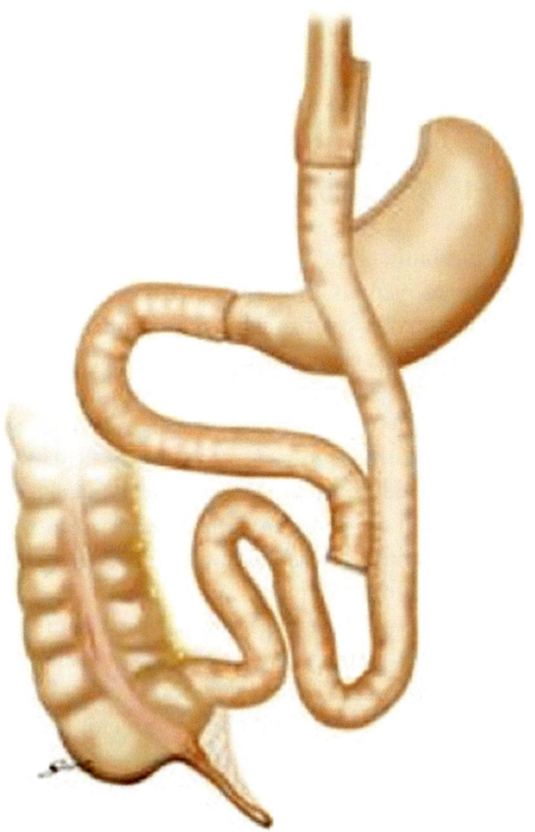

Fig. 6.1 Roux-en-Y Gastric Bypass

6.2 Position of the Patient

The position of the patient completely depends the surgeon's preference. Many surgeons prefer to use the split-leg position, but others prefer the

K. Kasama, MD, FACS
Weight Loss and Metabolic Surgery Center,
Yotsuya Medical Cube, 7-7 Nibancho,
Chiyoda-ku, Tokyo 102-0084, Japan
e-mail: kazukasama@gmail.com

S.H. Choi, K. Kasama (eds.), *Bariatric and Metabolic Surgery*,
DOI 10.1007/978-3-642-35591-2_6, © Springer-Verlag Berlin Heidelberg 2014

supine position. Almost all surgeons prefer reverse Trendelenburg position. We use the split-leg reverse Trendelenburg position; the camera assistant stands between the legs and the surgeon stands on the right side of the patient.

6.3 LRYGB Consists of These Manipulations

1. Trocar insertion
2. Jejunojejunostomy
3. Gastric pouch formation
4. Gastrojejunostomy
5. Others (including mesenteric closure, leak test)
   Sequential order may depend on surgeons' preference.

6.3.1 Trocar Insertion

For morbidly obese patients, it is very difficult to do "open method" for the first trocar insertion. Initial entry is performed without insufflation using a 10 mm non-bladed optical trocar system. Using a bladed optical trocar system may cause serious injury to the blood vessels and lead to major hemorrhage, so we avoid using a bladed trocar for the first port. The camera is placed at 2–3 cm left from the midline, 18 cm from the xiphoid. Three 12 mm ports are placed at (1) 10 cm from the midline and just beneath the costal margin, (2) 10 cm below that port, and (3) 3 cm right from the midline and 2 cm beneath the right costal margin. One 5 mm port is placed just below the xiphoid to put the lever retractor before formation of the gastric pouch (Fig. 6.2).

Close attention to the angle of entry of the ports can reduce the resistance of the abdominal wall to the instruments, allowing for a more precise and less fatiguing operation.

6.3.2 Jejunojejunostomy

The omentum is displaced cephalad to expose the ligament of Treitz (Fig. 6.3). The length of the biliopancreatic tract, which means the length from the ligament of Treitz, may be determined

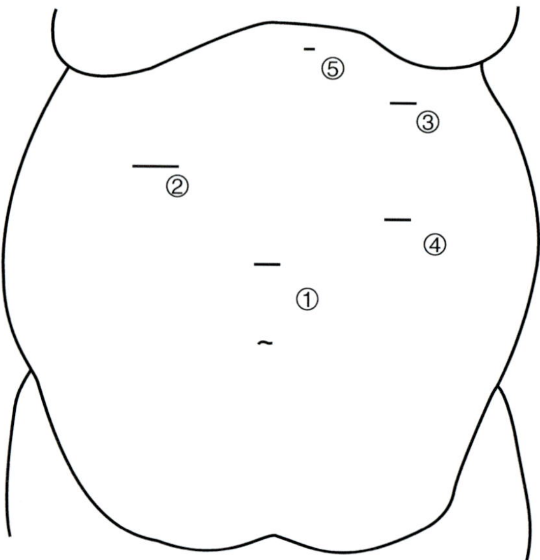

Fig. 6.2 Trocar position

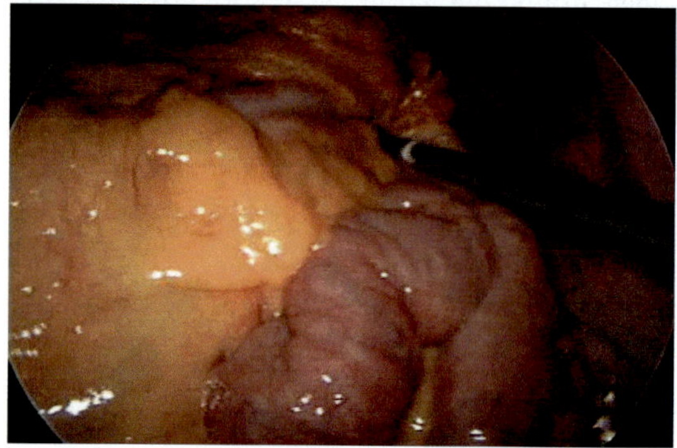

Fig. 6.3 Exposition of the ligament of Treits

by the surgeon's preference. Usually it is between 30 and 100 cm, and there is no uniform fashion for gastric bypass. The jejunum is transected with a white or camel cartridge linear stapler (Fig. 6.4), and the mesentery is divided with laparoscopic coagulating shears (LCS) including Harmonic Scalpel and SonoSurg (Fig. 6.5). Typically, the length of the Roux limb can be up to 200 cm without an associated increased incidence of malabsorptive complications. Jejunojejunostomy is performed with a side-to-side linear anastomosis using a white or camel cartridge linear stapler (Fig. 6.6), and the enterotomy is closed with a single layer of absorbable suture (Fig. 6.7). Some surgeons prefer to use a linear stapler to close the enterotomy, but this may cause stenosis. The

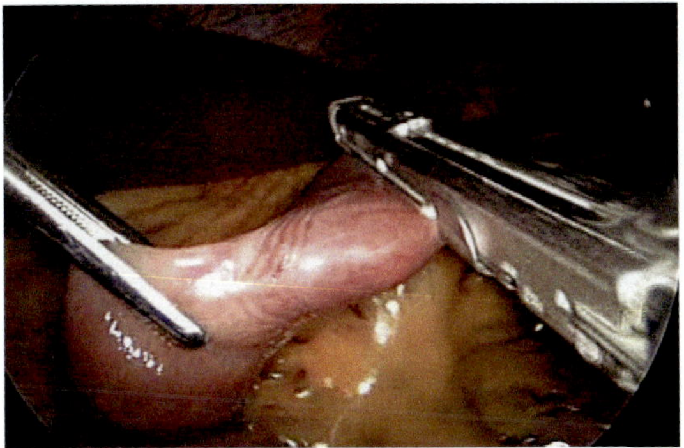

Fig. 6.4 Transection of jejunum

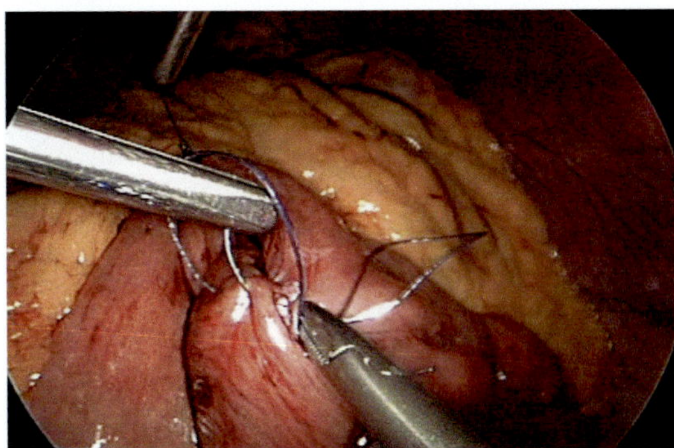

Fig. 6.7 Closure of the entry hole

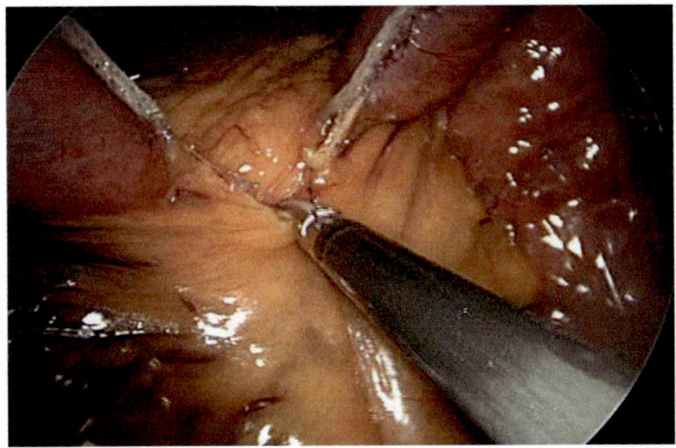

Fig. 6.5 Division of the mesentery

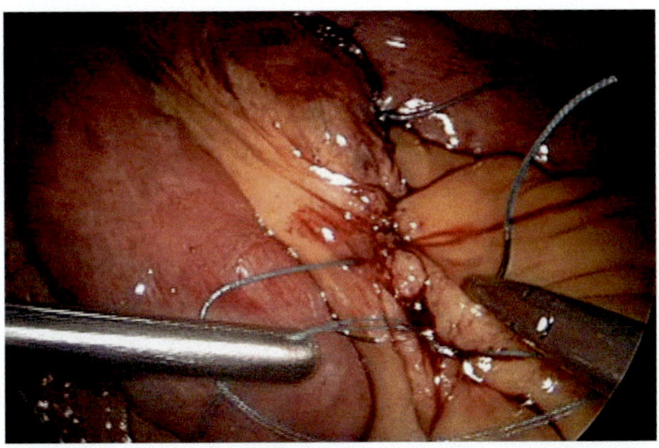

Fig. 6.8 Closure of the mesenteric defect

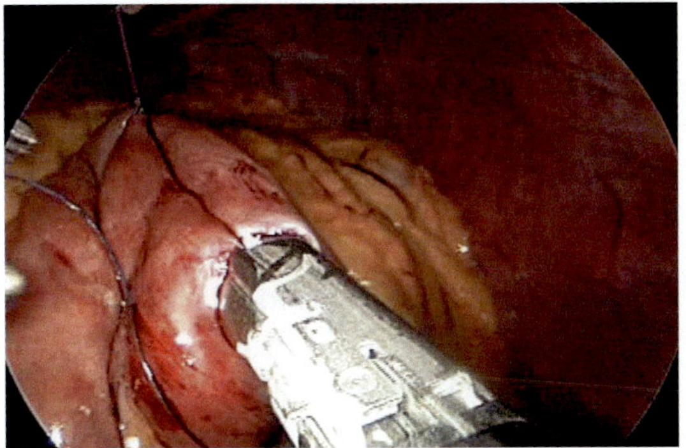

Fig. 6.6 Jejunojejunostomy

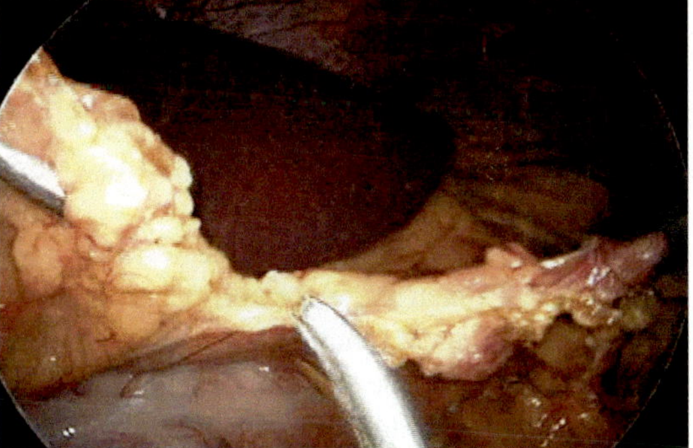

Fig. 6.9 Division of the omentum

mesenteric defect must be closed with a continuous, nonabsorbable suture to limit the possibility of an internal hernia (Fig. 6.8).

The Roux limb is passed in front of the transverse colon as is done in the "antecolic approach." To reduce the tension to the gastrojejunal anastomosis, the omentum should be divided with LCS (Fig. 6.9).

6.3.3   Gastric Pouch Formation

The liver retractor is placed before the pouch formation. Occasionally, a very large liver will not allow for sufficient visualization. It will be an indication for open conversion. Preoperative weight loss with a very low-calorie diet (VLCD)

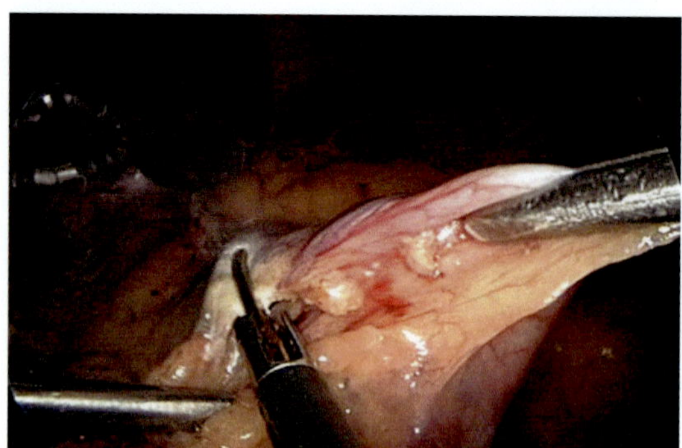

Fig. 6.10 Perigastric dissection

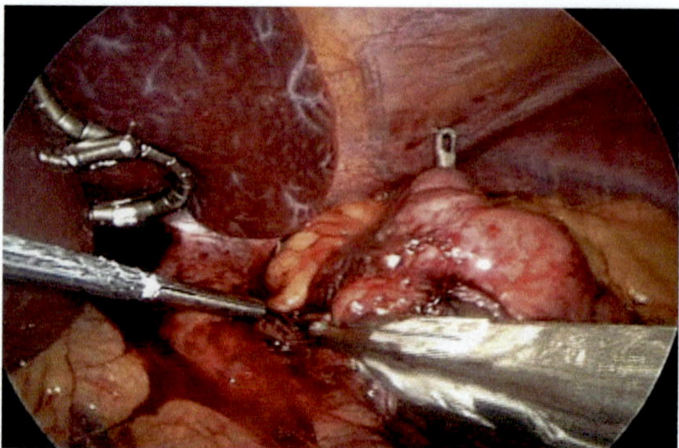

Fig. 6.12 Pouch formation with a 36 Fr tube

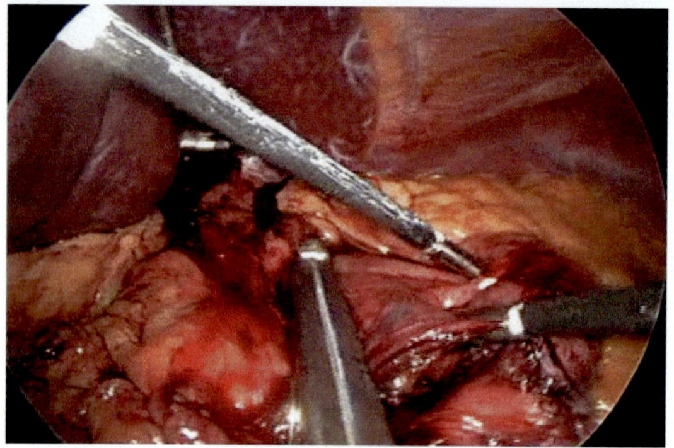

Fig. 6.11 Vertical application of the stapler

must be used before surgery to reduce the volume of the liver. Alternatively, the surgeon may decide to abort the procedure or to convert it to sleeve gastrectomy.

Perigastric dissection along the lesser curvature of the stomach is performed 5 cm distal to the gastroesophageal junction and continues until the retrogastric space is reached (Fig. 6.10). Dense adhesions to the pancreas will be encountered at this time. Care must be taken to avoid injury to the pancreas during adhesiolysis.

A blue or purple stapler is used to form the gastric pouch. It is essential to exclude the distended gastric fundus in order to maintain long-term weight loss. This requires meticulous dissection of the retrogastric space to the angle of His to avoid the injury of esophagus and spleen. A pouch volume of no more than 20 cc is optimal.

The inferior aspect of the pouch is determined with the first horizontal stapler from the right upper quadrant port. All subsequent firing is vertically oriented through the left port (Fig. 6.11). It is preferable to divide the fat pad at the hiatus to get better visualization of the angle of His prior to stapling.

A 36 Fr (12 mm) orogastric tube is inserted into the stomach after the first horizontal stapling assists in the estimation of pouch size and prevents inadvertent transection or impingement of staples on the esophagus (Fig. 6.12).

6.3.4 Gastrojejunostomy

Recently, antecolic reconstruction is more widely used than retrocolic reconstruction. As mentioned above, gastrojejunostomy is typically performed using one of three methods.

6.3.4.1 Circular Stapler Anastomosis (Fig. 6.13)

To use transoral circular stapler technique, the gastric pouch should be made bigger than that described above. A 25 mm circular stapler is used for the anastomosis.

The 16 Fr nasogastric tube is cut, and the tip of the anvil is attached to the cut end of the tube and tied to the tube. The nasogastric tube is passed with the anvil through the mouth and down the esophagus carefully, until the tip of the tube is seen to abut the pouch. A gastrostomy is made using LCS and the tip of the tube is pulled out. The excess tubing is then pulled out until the

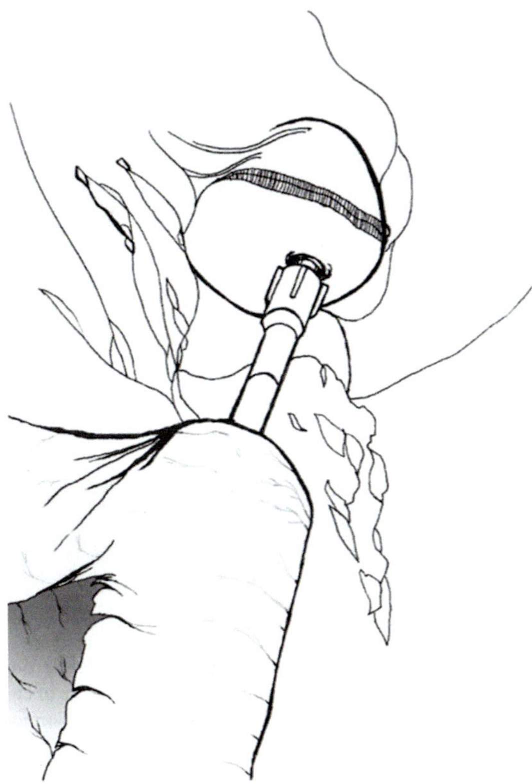

Fig. 6.13 Circular stapler anastomosis

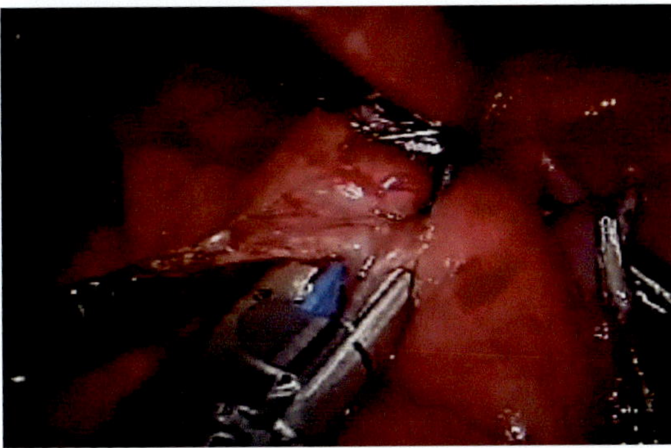

Fig. 6.14 Linear stapler anastomosis

metal tip of the anvil is seen exiting the pouch. The tube is completely removed from the anvil.

The staple line of the distal limb is opened using LSC. The left upper trocar is removed and the site is enlarged to accommodate the shaft of the circular stapler. The circular stapler is then passed transabdominally, intubated through an enterotomy into the Roux limb and used to retract the Roux limb upward toward the pouch. The white tip of the stapler is extended to perforate through the anti-mesenteric part of the Roux limb, and then removed. The stapler is connected to the anvil, closed and fired. The stapler is carefully brought out of the opening in the Roux limb and removed from the abdomen after engaging the wound protector. The end of the Roux limb is closed using the linear stapler.

6.3.4.2 Linear Stapler Anastomosis (Fig. 6.14)

This anastomosis technique is familiar to all surgeons because it is based on the side-to-side, functional end-to-end anastomosis. The linear stapler anastomosis technique involves a linear stapler to create the anastomosis, and the gastro-enteric opening used for the stapler insertion is closed either by a second application of a stapler or using the hand-sewn technique.

The gastric pouch is cleaned of overlying fat tissue posterior to the gastric staple line for the anastomosis. The Roux limb is sutured to the posterior wall of the pouch to reduce the tension to the stapler anastomosis. A controlled enterotomy is then made in the Roux limb with LCS, approximately 5 mm away from the suture line. Another controlled enterotomy is made in the adjacent posterior wall of the pouch. Placing the linear stapler into those openings is best facilitated by the first placing the larger jaw in the gastrostomy to dilate the opening appropriately and to develop a feel for the appropriate direction in which the stapler will pass without resistance. The stapler can be gently eased back and the smaller jaw is inserted to the enterotomy on the Roux limb. The jaws are advanced into the bowel to the 2.5 cm mark and then fired.

The closure of the gastroenterotomy is accomplished using running absorbable sutures in one or two layers over the stent.

Some surgeons prefer to use a stapler to close the gastroenterotomy to avoid intracorporeal suturing. Testing the anastomosis is recommended with an endoscope or methylene blue test.

6.3.4.3 Hand-Suturing Anastomosis

The formation of the gastrojejunostomy begins with a running posterior, exterior layer of 3-0 or

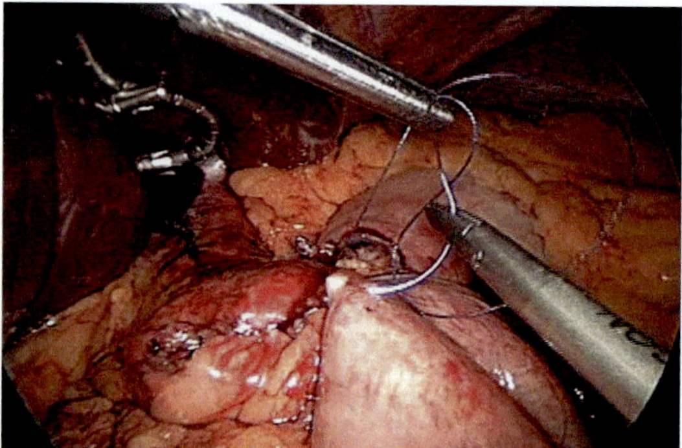

Fig. 6.15 Hand suturing anastomosis: the first layer

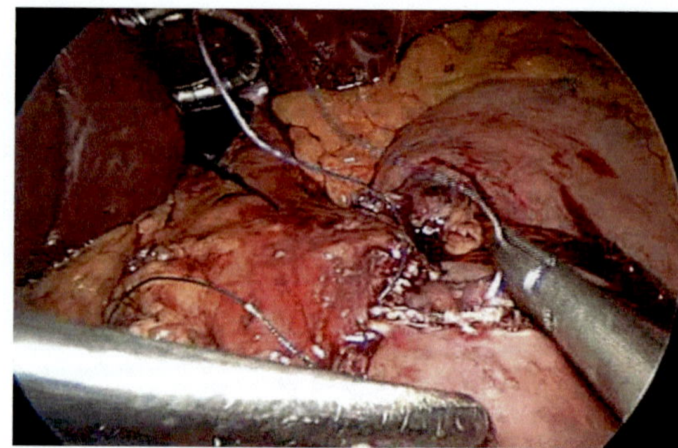

Fig. 6.17 Posterior full thickness layer suturing

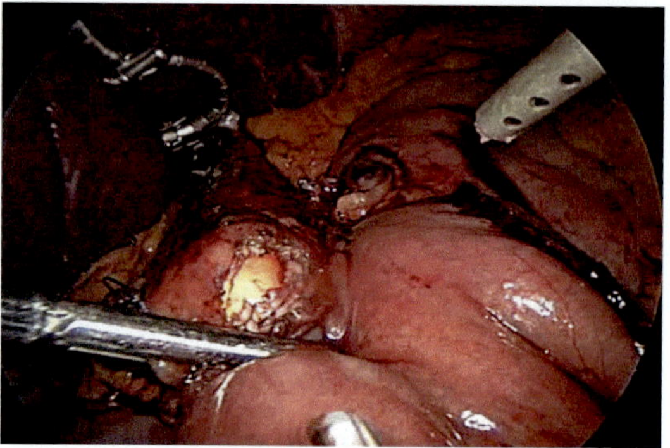

Fig. 6.16 Enterotomy on the pouch

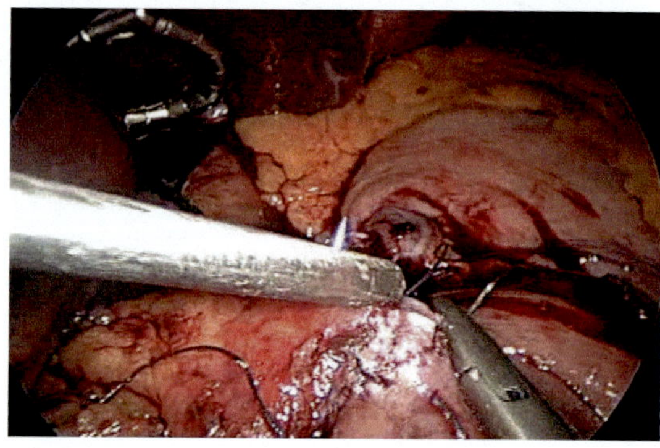

Fig. 6.18 Anterior full thickness layer suturing

2-0 absorbable sutures (Fig. 6.15). Beginning distally and sewing proximally, the anti-mesenteric side of the Roux limb is approximated to the inferior staple line of the gastric pouch, incorporating the staples in the suture line. Enterotomies are performed on the gastric pouch and the Roux limb adjacent to the suture line (Fig. 6.16). A second posterior, full thickness, running suture line is performed and continued anteriorly beyond the termination of the first posterior suture (Fig. 6.17).

Two anterior suture lines are run from the distal anterior aspect of the enterotomy, the first being full thickness (Fig. 6.18) and the second a seromuscular suture (Fig. 6.19). Prior to completion of the anastomosis, the 36 Fr orogastric tube is carefully inserted across the anastomosis to help calibrate the opening as well as to provide assurance of a patent anastomosis. The anterior

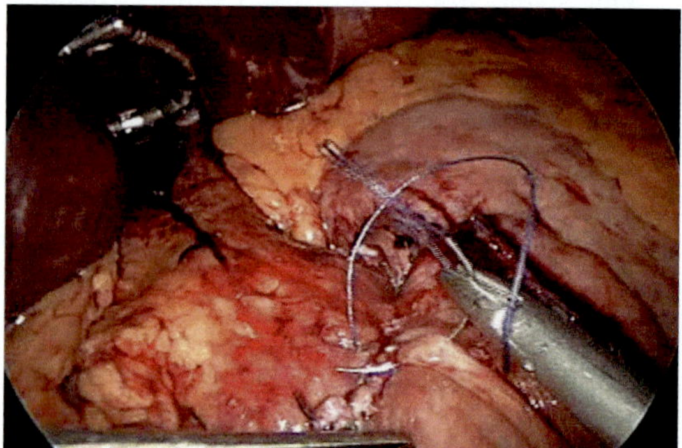

Fig. 6.19 Anterior seromuscular layer suturing

sutures are tied with their respective posterior counterparts.

The anastomosis and proximal staple lines can be tested with blue dye, air insufflation via the orogastric tube, or operative endoscopy.

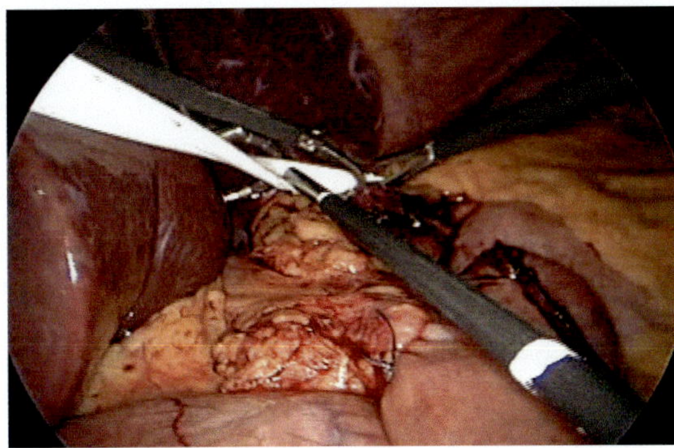

Fig. 6.20 Drain insertion

We routinely insert the drain, but its use depends on the surgeons' preference (Fig. 6.20).

We prefer to perform hand-sewn anastomosis. The advantages and disadvantages of using the hand-sewn technique are as follows:

Advantages

Low leak rate in "open" series

Less expensive than other techniques

Does not require enlargement of port or incur increased infections caused by contamination of port site

Allows for a small, longitudinal gastric pouch

Can be performed by a single surgeon without a skilled surgeon as an assistant

Allows surgeon to develop important skills necessary to resolve any complications

In my personal opinion, being a surgeon, the last one listed is the most important advantage of hand-sewn anastomosis.

Disadvantage

The only disadvantage is that there is a "long learning curve."

6.3.5   Others

In all three methods, a potential site of an internal hernia, including Petersen's space, should be closed with sutures.

The port sites are inspected for bleeding when the trocars are withdrawn, and the skin is closed with simple absorbable sutures.

6.4   Postoperative Management

Perioperative antibiotic is continued for 24 h, and thromboembolism prophylaxis continues until the patient starts walking. Analgesia is in the form of patient-controlled narcotic delivery systems and intravenous anti-inflammatory drugs. Oral and intravenous antiemetic agents are routinely used.

The patients are started on clear liquid at least on the first day after surgery, sometimes on the day of surgery, and are required to ambulate with assistance. Preoperative oral medications can be resumed as soon as the patients can tolerate clear liquid. Most of the patients can be discharged on the second postoperative day.

Patients are continued on a clear liquid diet for 1 week and slowly advanced to solids over a 3–4-week period. Patients are instructed to take a proton pump inhibitor for a month.

Routine follow-ups over the telephone are at 1 and 2 weeks, and routine follow-up visits are at the 1-month mark and quarterly for the first year, then every half a year for the second year and on a yearly basis after that. Ongoing nutritional, emotional, exercise counseling, and support groups are provided. Complete nutritional assessment occurs on a yearly basis or as dictated by symptoms or clinical suspicions.

Further Videos

Electronic supplementary material is available in the online version of this chapter at (doi:10.1007/978-3-642-35591-2_6) and accessible for authorised users. Videos can also be accessed at http://www.springerimages.com/videos/978-3-642-35590-5

References

1. Wittgrove AC, Clark GW, Tremblay LJ. Laparoscopic gastric bypass, Roux-en-Y: preliminary report of five cases. Obes Surg. 1994;4(4):353–7.
2. Buchwald H, Oien DM. Metabolic/bariatric surgery worldwide 2011. Obes Surg. 2013;23(4):427–36.

Joo Ho Lee and Do Joong Park

7.1 Introduction

Sleeve gastrectomy (SG) is a vertical left gastrectomy of the body and fundus to create a long, narrow tubular gastric sleeve along the lesser curvature that reduces the size of gastric reservoir to 80–120 ml (Fig. 7.1). SG was originally intended as a bridge procedure for high-risk super obese patients preceding the definitive bariatric procedure such as biliopancreatic diversion with duodenal switch (BPD/DS) or Roux-en-Y gastric bypass (RYGB). However, the initial promising results of SG in terms of weight loss and resolution of comorbidities have rendered it popular not only as a first-stage procedure but also as a primary bariatric surgery. Laparoscopic sleeve gastrectomy (LSG) is now considered as a newer stand-alone operation being performed with increasing frequency, which is approved by

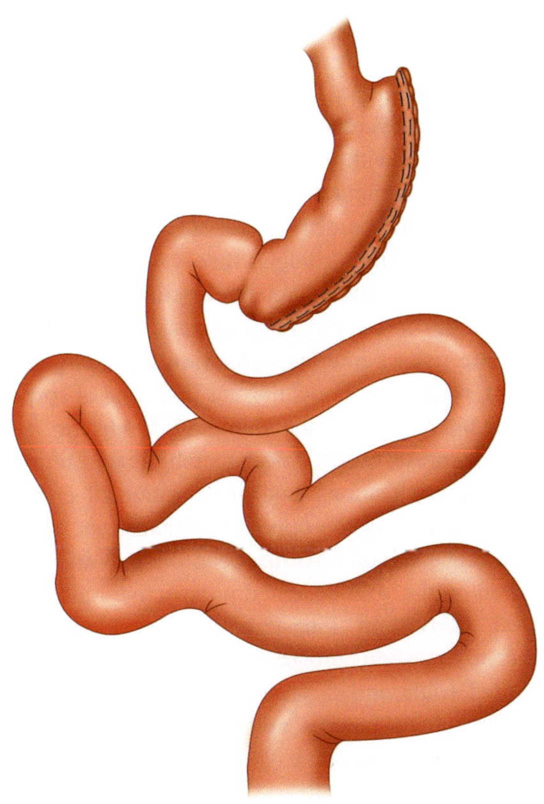

Fig. 7.1 Illustration of sleeve gastrectomy

J.H. Lee, MD (✉)
Department of Surgery, Ewha Womans University
School of Medicine, Seoul, Korea
e-mail: gsljh@ewha.ac.kr

D.J. Park, MD
Department of Surgery, Seoul National University
College of Medicine, Seoul, Korea
e-mail: djpark@snubh.org

both the American Society for Metabolic and Bariatric Surgery (ASMBS) and the American College of Surgeons (ACS). In 2011, it occupied over 25 % of bariatric procedures worldwide, which became the second most commonly performed bariatric procedure after RYGB. While

S.H. Choi, K. Kasama (eds.), *Bariatric and Metabolic Surgery*,
DOI 10.1007/978-3-642-35591-2_7, © Springer-Verlag Berlin Heidelberg 2014

the mechanism of action seen after SG is mainly regarded as restriction of calorie intake, the hormonal changes related to gastric resection and expedited food transport to distal small bowel might be involved as well. Ghrelin is a hunger-regulating peptide hormone mainly produced from the fundus of the stomach. Besides its well-known function in modulating appetite, ghrelin may directly regulate glucose homeostasis. Although the effect of ghrelin to incretins remains unclear, it has been suggested that the low levels of ghrelin after surgery are attributable to the secretion of endogenous gastrointestinal hormones such as GLP-1 and PYY that stimulate pancreatic beta cells. The pattern of rapid gastric emptying could be another factor that influences diabetes resolution. Rapid meal emptying into small intestine could contribute to shorter contact time of food with proximal gut and rapid arrival of food to terminal ileum. As a consequence, the hormonal environment of diabetes patients could be ameliorating (hindgut theory). It also has advantages including relatively simple surgical technique, no intestinal anastomosis thus excluding the risk of internal herniation and marginal ulcer, no foreign body, normal intestinal absorption, prevention of the dumping syndrome by pylorus preservation, fewer metabolic and nutritional complications, and preservation of endoscopic access to the upper gastrointestinal tract. The drawback of LSG has been the lack of data based on the well-designed prospective randomized study and long-term results. However, recently several prospective randomized controlled trials and 5 years or more of midterm results about laparoscopic sleeve gastrectomy proved this procedure is safe, effective, and durable.

Although the procedure is technically simple, its complications such as staple line leak can be very serious and difficult to treat, even life threatening. Lack of technical standardization will result in poor outcomes. With the surgeons' required technical experiences and knowledge, the standardization of procedure is mandatory for the excellent outcome of this procedure. However, there is so far no standardization in surgical techniques regarding sizing the sleeve, the first and last firing sites, staple line reinforcement, and so on.

7.2 Indications

The general indication of sleeve gastrectomy for morbid obesity is similar to that of gastric banding or LRYGB:

1. Body mass index (BMI) >40 kg/m^2 or BMI >35 kg/m^2 with significant comorbidities
2. BMI >37 kg/m^2 or BMI >32 kg/m^2 with significant comorbidities (Asia-Pacific)
3. Failed attempts at nonsurgical weight loss
   However, specific considerations can be posed to selection of sleeve gastrectomy.

- First procedure in staged surgery in high-risk patients:
  1. Super-super-obese patients (BMI >60 kg/m^2)
  2. Morbidly obese patients with significant comorbidity such as liver cirrhosis, Crohn's disease, multiple sclerosis, or rheumatoid arthritis
- Primary bariatric surgery:
  1. Lower BMI
  2. Adolescent or elderly morbidly obese patients
  3. Gastric lesions: Helicobacter pylori infection, ulcer, and chronic atrophic gastritis
  4. Desire to undergo a relatively simple restrictive operation not requiring the placement of a foreign body
  5. Necessity to continue specific medication (immunosuppressant, anti-inflammatory)
  6. Revisional surgery after gastric banding failure

Sleeve gastrectomy may be contraindicated in patients with:

1. Severe gastroesophageal reflux disease or large hiatal hernia
2. Barrett's esophagus
3. Ulcer located in the lesser curvature of the stomach
4. Common relative contraindicated patients for LRYGB

7.3 Surgical Technique

7.3.1 General Setting

The general settings such as anesthesia, surgical team, and instruments for laparoscopic sleeve gastrectomy are similar to those described in the "basic techniques and instruments."

7.3.2 Patient Position

Under general anesthesia, patient is positioned in reverse Trendelenburg position with slight left side up to facilitate operative field exposure. Urinary catheter and sequential compression devices are placed. Generally the operator stands at the right side of the patient with the camera operator and the first assistant at the left side with scrub nurse.

7.3.3 Port Placement

Introduction of first trocar to creating pneumoperitoneum is one of the most critical procedures which can be lethal during bariatric surgery. There are three methods:
1. Use of Veress needle
2. Open method
3. Use of visual trocar

A transparent trocar is used, through which a camera tip can be inserted. The trocar and zero-degree camera are inserted simultaneously through the abdominal wall under laparoscopic view of abdominal wall layers.

CO_2 gas is insufflated to create pneumoperitoneum to set the intra-abdominal pressure approximately 15 mmHg.

Generally the number of ports can be variable from five to six ports. Recently some surgeons try to perform the procedure using single incision or through the vagina (NOTES). It usually depends on the degree of patient obesity and surgeon's preference. The location and size of ports are also different from cases to cases. The usual port placement is illustrated in Fig. 7.2.

7.3.4 Liver Retraction

In order to get a good exposure around gastroesophageal junction, effective liver retraction is critical. Restricted calorie intake for at least 2 weeks before surgery may reduce left lateral segment volume of the liver. Several methods are

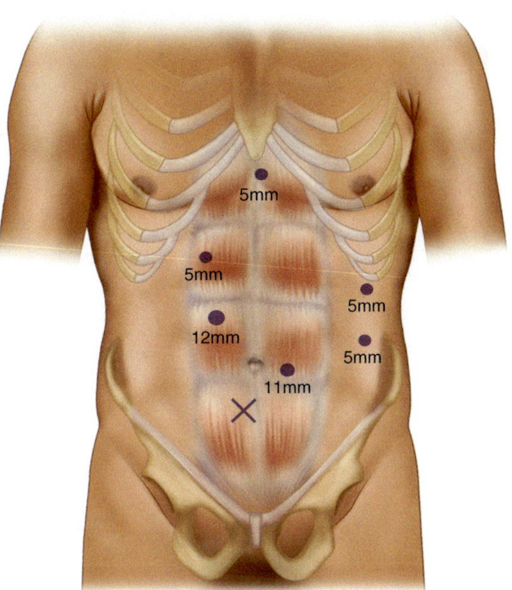

Fig. 7.2 Port placement (six ports)

used to retract the liver. Three-finger or five-finger liver retractor, snake retractor, or Nathanson liver retractor is frequently used. Suture technique is also available, but it is hard to apply to super obese patients.

7.3.5 Laparoscopic Sleeve Gastrectomy

7.3.5.1 Starting the Dissection of the Greater Curvature

The pylorus is identified. The starting point of future stapling should be 2–8 cm away from the pylorus, and it should be marked beforehand (Fig. 7.3). It is easy to make the first window between the stomach and greater omentum at a slight proximal site away from the starting point (Fig. 7.4). The distal stomach is grasped and pulled to the right and upper, and then the greater omentum is spread to the counter-direction. Ultrasonic coagulating shears (e.g., Harmonic Scalpel™) or vessel-sealing system (e.g., LigaSure) is useful to divide small vascular arcades of great omentum from the greater curvature of the stomach. Dissection is continued to get approach to short gastric vessels near the lower pole of the spleen.

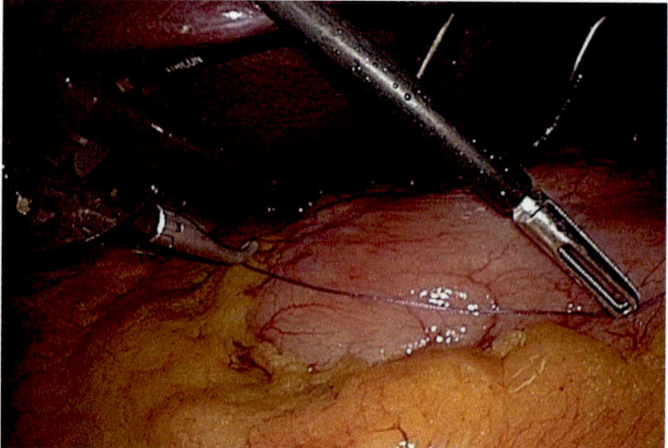

Fig. 7.3 Starting point is measured about 4–5 cm away from the pylorus

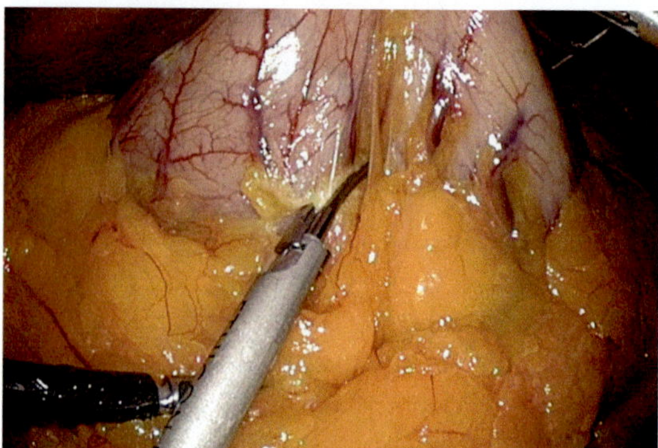

Fig. 7.4 Dissection begins by making a window at a transparent area between arcade and it is easier to start dissection from the proximal to the marking point

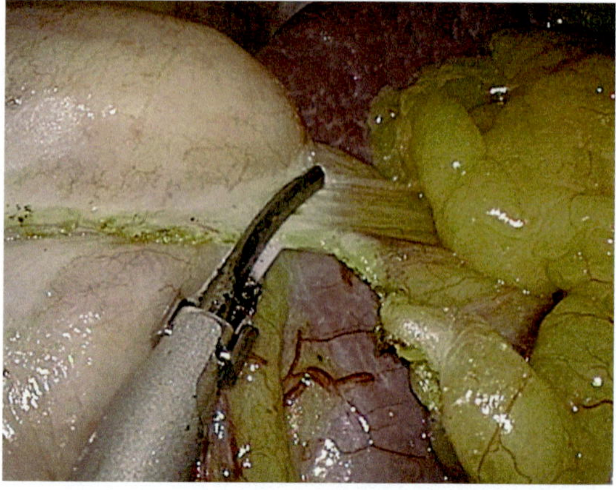

Fig. 7.5 Short gastric vessel division close to gastric wall. Tension between the fundus and spleen should be minimized to prevent splenic tear

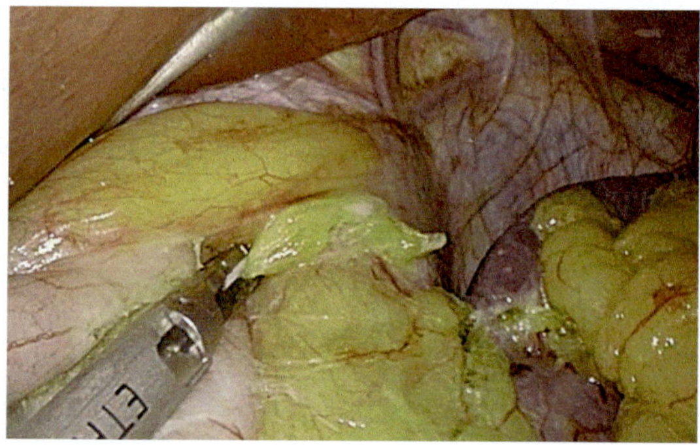

Fig. 7.6 Left diaphragmatic crus should be exposed for the complete removal of gastric fundus

7.3.5.2 Mobilization of the Fundus

The short gastric vessels should be divided near to the gastric wall carefully with least tension between the stomach and spleen. Otherwise, bleeding with spleen capsule tearing may occur (Fig. 7.5). All division must be carried out under direct vision, not by blind or blunt dissection. The gastrophrenic ligament should be incised to ensure complete mobilization of fundus. The dissection is continued to the point of His angle and left diaphragmatic crus (Fig. 7.6). Sometimes, removal of fat pad around gastroesophageal junction may facilitate the exposure of left crus. Pulling the dissected fundus to the right and cranial and taking down the greater omentum to the left would make it easy to expose and dissect His angle area. Detachment of the posterior adhesion between the stomach and pancreas is important in order to remove the fundus completely and to make a good gastric tube having even anterior and posterior gastric wall (Fig. 7.7). However, too much mobilization might cause a twist of the gastric tube later. One should pay attention not to injure the blood vessels on lesser curvature including left gastric artery. The presence of hiatal hernia should be assessed, and if present the hiatus should be repaired.

7.3.5.3 Transection of the Stomach

After full mobilization of the stomach, gastric division is performed using a laparoscopic linear stapler from the antrum toward the angle of His. The first stapling for thick antrum to incisura angularis of the stomach should be cautious to

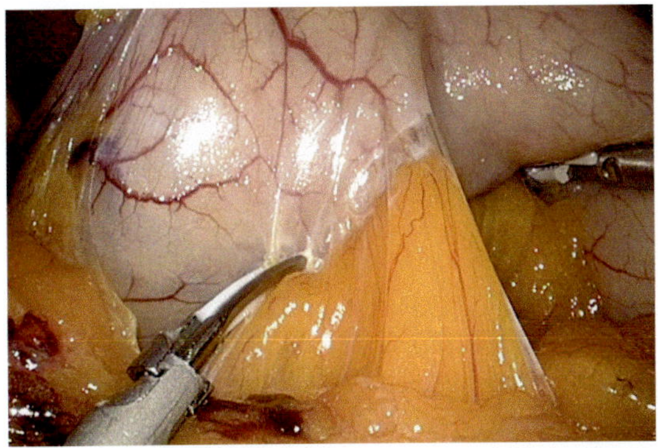

Fig. 7.7 Posterior adhesion should be detached in order to make a good sleeve

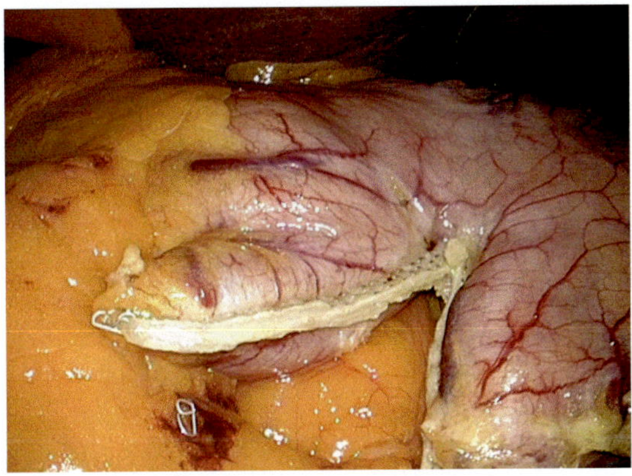

Fig. 7.9 Staple line after the first stapling

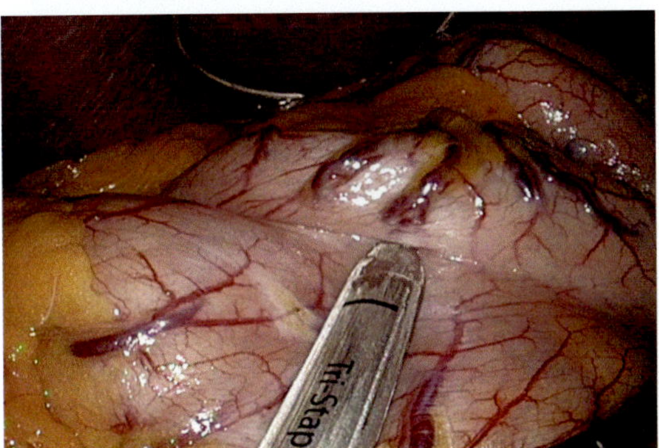

Fig. 7.8 First staple is ready to fire

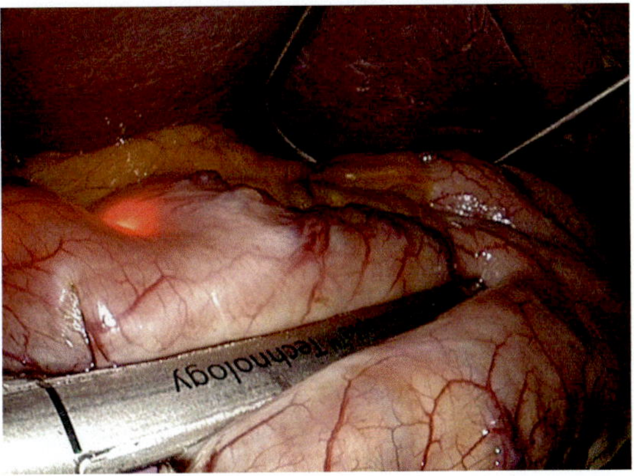

Fig. 7.10 Gastroscopy can be used as a bougie during transection of the stomach

avoid stricture. The height of staple cartridge is important in the transection of the stomach. Too narrow staple cartridge can cause an ischemia which leads to a possible leak, while too wide cartilage can cause postoperative bleeding. Usually stapling of the gastric antrum should be performed with green cartilage (closed heights 2.0 mm, 4.8/60 mm) followed by with sequential blue cartilage for the remaining corpus and fundus (closed height 1.5 mm 3.5/60 mm, blue). Some surgeons recommend compression for 10–20 s before firing. A bendable (reticulating) linear stapler is useful to transect the stomach efficiently.

Before and/or after the first firing of the distal part of the stomach (Figs. 7.8 and 7.9), the use of bougie is strongly recommended to calibrate sleeve size to prevent any constriction or injury of GE junction (Fig. 7.10). The stapler is fired consecutively along the bougie to His angle. When stapling, one should stretch the stomach by pulling the greater curvature side of the stomach laterally in order to make a well-lineated staple line and good-shaped gastric tube (Fig. 7.11). Placing the last staple should be parallel to the left diaphragmatic crus not to injure the esophagus (Fig. 7.12). Reinforcement along the staple line with seroserous invaginating running suture is performed to control bleeding and reduce the risk of leak (Fig. 7.13). One can perform leakage test by infusing methylene blue, air insufflations, or intraoperative endoscopy. Specimen is inserted into a plastic bag and extracted out of the abdominal cavity through the largest port wound or by slightly extending one port wound (Fig. 7.14). One drain may be inserted along the staple line.

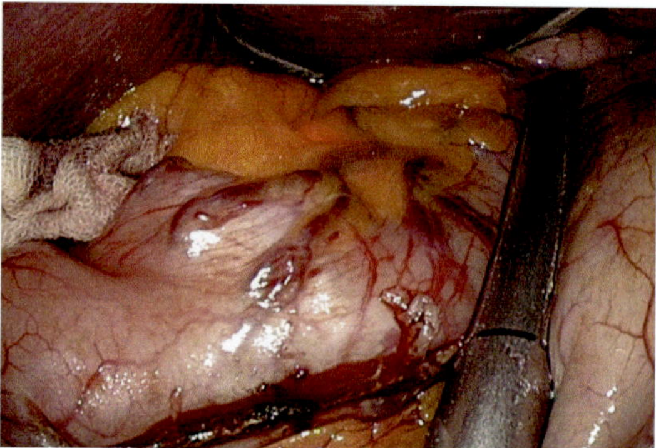

Fig. 7.11 Continue transection of the stomach being parallel to the lesser curvature of the stomach

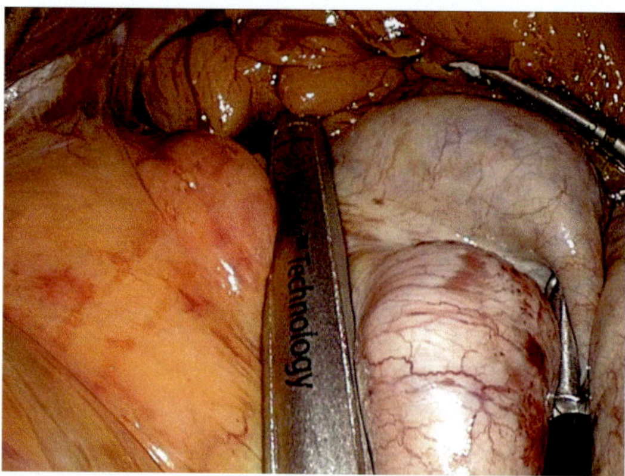

Fig. 7.12 Last firing should be performed away from a His angle and be parallel to the esophagus

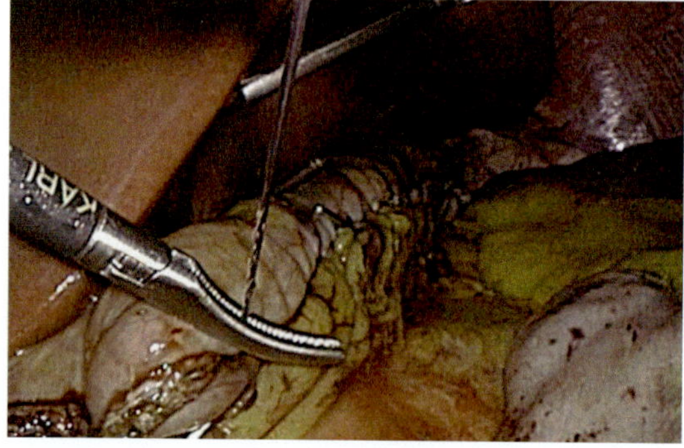

Fig. 7.13 Staple line along the gastric sleeve

Some surgeons prefer the so-called medial to lateral approach, in which the stapling of the stomach is done just after creating a small window enough to insert a linear stapler before full mobilization of the stomach.

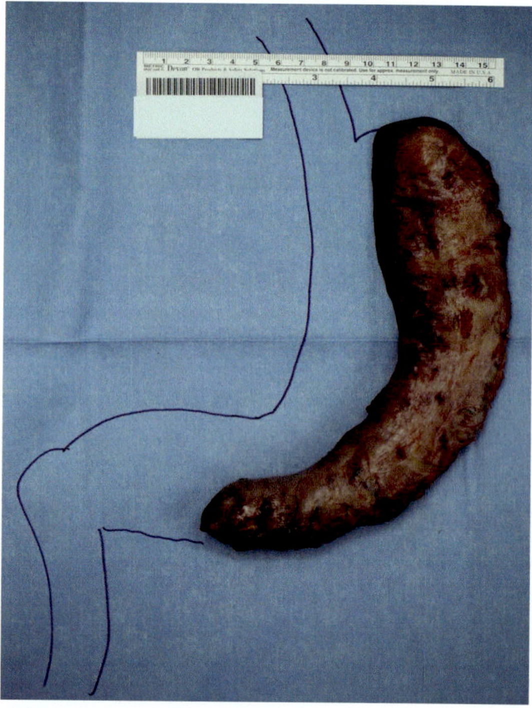

Fig. 7.14 Specimen is extracted out of the abdomen through a port wound

7.4 Complications and Management

LSG is regarded to be positioned between the LRYGB and LAGB in the overall morbidity and mortality rate, which ranged 2.0–12.0 % and 0.1–0.5 %, respectively. The most prevalent complications after SG are leak, bleeding, stricture, and gastroesophageal reflux.

7.4.1 Leak

Staple line leak is the most dreaded complication, reported 0–8 % incidence after LSG. The most frequent leak point is near the gastroesophageal junction. Because of the lack of adequately powered randomized controlled study, it is impossible to suggest definitely the factor leading to a leak. The high intragastric pressure from small sleeve size, compromised blood supply, failure of staple device, and stricture or torsion of incisura angularis might be some of the causes of leak.

Symptoms are tachycardia, fever, abdominal pain, or left shoulder pain. Radiologic study such as CT scan or upper GI contrast series can be helpful, though not always positive. Most minor leaks can be solved by conservative management such as nothing per oral with parenteral nutrition, antibiotics, or percutaneous drainage. Endoscopic clipping, self-expanding retrievable stent insertion, or fibrin/cyanoacrylate sealant can be applied to the patients whose leaks are not solved by conservative management. If the patient is hemodynamically unstable or septic, immediate laparoscopic or open reoperative drainage procedure should be performed. Oversewing at the leak point usually fails to heal. Roux-en-Y gastric bypass or total gastrectomy may be required for a long-standing refractory leak.

7.4.2 Bleeding

The incidence of staple line bleeding has been reported to be 0–8.7 %. Bleeding may come from gastroepiploic arcade, a tearing of the spleen, or staple line. To prevent gastroepiploic arcade bleeding, dissection begins from the transparent window very close to the greater curvature of the stomach, and ultrasonic coagulating shears or vessel-sealing system should be used. One should not perform blunt dissection and, instead, should make a small hole first with laparoscopic dissector and then cut the vessel with energy device under direct vision. Escaping from much tension between the stomach and spleen is important to avoid tearing the spleen. Reinforcement or buttress material may be helpful to prevent staple line bleeding.

7.4.3 Stricture

The incidence of stricture is reported to be 0–5.0 %. The small bougie size could be the cause; incisura angularis is the greatest potential site. Balloon dilatation or stent insertion can be applied to a stricture after sleeve gastrectomy. For a long-segment stricture, laparoscopic sero-myotomy may be helpful. Conversion to Roux-en-Y gastric bypass might be needed to treat further refractory stenosis.

7.4.4 Gastroesophageal Reflux Disease (GERD)

Incidence of gastroesophageal reflux disease (GERD) after sleeve gastrectomy was reported to be 6.5–40 %. SG is regarded to induce or exacerbate GERD in general, although there is a debate regarding whether SG induces or treats GERD. Decreasing in lower esophageal sphincter pressure (LESP) from disruption of phrenoesophageal ligament, partial resection of sling fibers could be the cause of GERD. The narrow sleeve (high intragastric pressure), smaller antrum, and stricture of incisura angularis could be the other causes. In contrast, accelerated gastric emptying, decreased intra-abdominal pressure, and decreased acid production from fundus removal might attribute to improve GERD. One should identify whether the patient has hiatal hernia or not, both preoperatively and intraoperatively. Most surgeons recommend the approximation of the crura if hiatal hernia is found during LSG. Dissection to the posterior is necessary to inspect and repair the hiatal hernia. Preservation of antrum for rapid gastric emptying might be helpful to prevent GERD. Proton pump inhibitor is helpful to resolve the symptom. For a severe, refractory GERD, Roux-en-Y gastric bypass may be necessary.

7.5 Controversy in Surgical Techniques

Although LSG is newly accepted as a safe and effective bariatric procedure, there are so far many technical controversies regarding bougie size, distance from pylorus where the first staple firing, staple line reinforcement, section near GE junction, and the use of intraoperative leakage test. Standardization of surgical technique is indispensable for improving effectiveness and minimalizing complication rate. According to the Third International Consensus Summit on Sleeve Gastrectomy in December 2010, the mean size of used bougie was 36 Fr (28–60 F), mean distance from pylorus to start resection was 4.8 cm (1.5–7.0 cm), 67.1 % of surgeons perform staple line reinforcement (57 % buttress material, 43 %

oversewing), and 95 % of fundus is excised (a tiny portion is maintained lateral to the angle of His).

7.5.1 Bougie Size

Although there is still no general agreement regarding optimal bougie size, there has been a trend toward the use of smaller diameter of bougie for more effective restriction and sustained weight loss. For SG works as an effective restrictive procedure in a long term, the size of sleeve should be tighter as much as possible. However, the tighter the sleeve, the higher the intragastric pressure, and consequently the greater the incidence of leak. In other words, there is an inverse relationship between size of bougie in diameter and rate of leak.

According to a systematic review and meta-analysis of 112 studies with 9991 patients, the overall leak incidence was 2.2 % and the bougie size was the only significant prognostic factor. The mean bougie size used was 38.2 ± 6.4 Fr. Utilizing bougie size more than 40 Fr decreases leak without impacting weight loss up to 3 years. Although it is inconclusive, the optimal bougie size should be more than 40 Fr for decreasing risk of leak and less than 50 Fr for effective and sustained restrictive function based on the available evidences so far.

7.5.2 Staple Line Reinforcement

Several surgical techniques have been proposed to reduce the risk of staple line leak and bleeding. Whether these techniques have any impact for reducing the risk is still controversial, and the randomized trial to definitely estimate the effectiveness of each technique might be impossible. Lots of surgeons prefer reinforcement of the staple line by using reinforcing material such as buttress stapler, seroserous suture invagination (or through-and-through suture), or biological sealants to minimalize the possibility of bleeding and leak. According to the meta-analysis with 1,335 participants of two RCTs and six cohort studies,

reinforcing the staple line (buttress or oversewing) seemed to reduce the risk of leak and reinforcement with a buttress materials seemed to reduce the risk of bleeding, although not statistically significant.

Some surgeons prefer not to perform any reinforcement procedure because it has no effect. In addition, buttress material is expensive, and oversewing sometimes could lead to stricture of sleeve or be the cause of leak or bleeding from tissue tears caused by the suture. However, the number of cases of currently available data is too small to be conclusive; more than 10,000 procedures would be needed to reach the statistical significant result.

7.5.3 The Distance From Pylorus to Start Distal Resection

The starting point of transection is controversial. The consensus of the first firing point is 2–8 cm from the pylorus. Some surgeons reserve antrum intact in order not to disturb gastric emptying and decreasing intragastric pressure which may be the cause of proximal leak. But, the others concern about the weight regain from sleeve dilatation after long-term follow-up and recommend resecting close to the pylorus to restrict food intake more and induce better weight reduction.

7.5.4 Proximal Section of the Stomach

The most frequent leak point is near the gastroesophageal junction. Regarding the last firing near the His angle, there is a controversy about proper transection line. One of the proposed causes of proximal leak is vascular theory. For complete mobilization of fundus, the blood vessels of posterolateral side of gastroesophageal junction (the short gastric vessels, posterior gastric artery, and left inferior phrenic artery) should be completely divided. Therefore, the lateral side of gastroesophageal junction (angle of His area) becomes the most poorly vascularized critical area. It is usually recommended to stay away from gastroesophageal junction leaving 1–2 cm of gastric remnant during the last fire in order to prevent a possible leak. Some surgeons recommend to leave "dog ear" at the His angle. However, the other surgeons prefer transection just next to the His angle not to retain any remnant fundus which may dilate and cause weight regain in the long-term follow-up.

Conclusion

According to the worldwide survey in 2011, there was a marked increase in LSG with a concomitant steep decline in LAGB over the past 8 years. Although LSG is now considered as a newer stand-alone operation being performed with increasing frequency for its proven safety and midterm efficacy, its surgical techniques need to be standardized. With the surgeons' required technical experiences and knowledge, the standardization of procedure is mandatory for the excellent outcome of this procedure. Through the technical standardization, we can search for the most optimal size of sleeve and most effective reinforcement method for the long stapler line, which would result in the substantial and durable weight loss with minimal risk of complications.

Further Videos

Electronic supplementary material is available in the online version of this chapter at (doi:10.1007/978-3-642-35591-2_7) and accessible for authorised users. Videos can also be accessed at http://www.springerimages.com/videos/978-3-642-35590-5

Further Reading

Brethauer SA, Hammel JP, Schauer PR. Systematic review of sleeve gastrectomy as staging and primary bariatric procedure. Surg Obes Relat Dis. 2009;5(4): 469–75.

Buchwald H. Bariatric surgery: a systematic review and meta-analysis. JAMA. 2004;292:1724–37.

Buchwald H, Estok R, Fahrbach K, et al. Weight and type 2 diabetes after bariatric surgery: systematic review and meta analysis. Am J Med. 2009;122(3):248–56.e5.

Buchwald H, Oien DM. Metabolic/bariatric surgery Worldwide 2008. Obes Surg. 2009;19(12):1605–11.

Buchwald H, Oien DM. Metabolic/bariatric surgery worldwide 2011. Obes Surg. 2013;23(4):427–36.

Akkary E, Duffy A, Bell R. Deciphering the sleeve: technique, indications, efficacy, and safety of sleeve gastrectomy. Obes Surg. 2008;18:1323–9.

Gagner M, Deitel M, Kalberer TL, Erickson AL, Crosby RD. The second international consensus summit for sleeve gastrectomy, March 19–21, 2009. Surg Obes Relat Dis. 2009;5(4):476–85.

Himpens J, Dapri G, Cadiere GB. A prospective randomized study between laparoscopic gastric banding and laparoscopic isolated sleeve gastrectomy: results after 1 and 3 years. Obes Surg. 2006;16: 1450–6.

Himpens J, Dobbeleir J, Peeters G. Long-term results of laparoscopic sleeve gastrectomy for obesity. Ann Surg. 2010;252:319–24.

Braghetto I, Lanzarini E, Korn O, Valladares H, Molina JC, Henriquez A. Manometric changes of the lower esophageal sphincter after sleeve gastrectomy in obese patients. Obes Surg. 2010;20:357–62.

Langer FB, Reza Hoda MA, Bohdjadian A, Felberbauer FX, Zacherl J, Wenzl E, et al. Sleeve gastrectomy and gastric banding: effects on plasma ghrelin levels. Obes Surg. 2005;15(7):1024–9.

Ferrer-Márquez M, Belda-Lozano R, Ferrer-Ayza M. Technical controversies in laparoscopic sleeve gastrectomy. Obes Surg. 2012;22:182–7.

Gagner M. Leaks after sleeve gastrectomy are associated with smaller bougies prevention and treatment strategies. Surg Laparosc Endosc Percutan Tech. 2010;20(3):166–9.

Parikh M, Issa R, McCrillis A, Saunders JK, Ude-Welcome A, Gagner M. Surgical strategies that may decrease leak after laparoscopic sleeve gastrectomy: a systematic review and meta-analysis of 9991 cases. Ann Surg. 2013;257(2):231–7.

Peterli R, Wolnerhanssen B, Peters T, et al. Improvement in glucose metabolism after bariatric surgery: comparison of laparoscopic Roux-en-Y gastric bypass and laparoscopic sleeve gastrectomy: a prospective randomized trial. Ann Surg. 2009;250:234–41.

Rosenthal RJ, for the International Sleeve Gastrectomy Expert Panel. International Sleeve Gastrectomy Expert Panel Consensus Statement: best practice guidelines based on experience of >12,000 cases. Surg Obes Relat Dis. 2012;8:8–19.

Woelnerhanssen B, Peterli R, Steinert RE, Peters T, Borbely Y, Beglinger C. Effects of post bariatric surgery weight loss on adipokines and metabolic parameters: comparison of laparoscopic Roux-en-Y gastric bypass and laparoscopic sleeve gastrectomy-a prospective randomized trial. Surg Obes Relat Dis. 2011;7:561–8.

Victorzon M. An update on sleeve gastrectomy. Minerva Chir. 2012;67(2):153–63.

Choi YY, Bae J, Hur KY, Choi D, Kim YJ. Reinforcing the staple line during laparoscopic sleeve gastrectomy: does it have advantages? A meta-analysis. Obes Surg. 2012;22:1206–13.

Laparoscopic Adjustable Gastric Banding (LAGB)

8

Seong Min Kim

8.1 Introduction

Obesity has reached epidemic proportions worldwide and is often associated with metabolic disorders, such as type 2 diabetes, hypertension, and dyslipidemia, which increase the risk of cardiovascular disease. Bariatric surgery is known to be the most effective and long-lasting treatment for obesity and its comorbidities. Laparoscopic adjustable gastric banding (LAGB) is a minimally invasive operation that is being performed increasingly since it was introduced in the early 1990s. In Asia/Pacific, LAGB held steady from 2003 (80.4 %) to 2008 (82.5 %) and then fell in 2011 (32.6 %) [1]. However, considering the number of the LAGB performed in private clinic, it is still one of the most frequently performed bariatric procedures for morbid obesity. It is a safe procedure, easy to perform, reversible, and effective. Unlike other bariatric surgical procedures such as sleeve gastrectomy or gastric bypass, which alter the anatomy of the alimentary tract, LAGB is essentially a restrictive procedure that limits food capacity. These limits can be adjusted by injecting saline into the band system through a reservoir port, which alters the stoma diameter. With the adequately adjusted stoma, patients fitted with gastric band can be satisfied with small amount of nutritious food and resulting weight loss. A systematic review shows substantial and similar long-term weight losses for LAGB and other bariatric procedures [2]. Although minor (access port, pouch, infection) and major (slippage, erosion) complications of LAGB are increasingly reported recently, proper surgical technique and intensive patient education with good aftercare program can minimize the incidence of these complications.

8.2 Eligibility/Candidate for LAGB

Patients in our clinic are selected for LAGB procedure according to recent recommendations for use of Bariatric and Gastrointestinal Metabolic Surgery for Treatment of Obesity in the Asian Population [3] (Fig. 8.1). Patients with extreme age (<18 or >65 years), BMI below 30 kg/m², untreated major depression, drug or alcohol abuse, schizophrenia, previous surgery of esophagogastric junction, malignancy, and connective tissue disease were excluded as a candidate for LAGB. Some individuals have end-stage organ dysfunction of the heart, lungs, or both; they are unlikely to gain the benefit of longevity and improved health. Prader-Willi syndrome is another absolute contraindication because no surgical therapy affects the constant need to eat by these patients.

S.M. Kim, MD, PhD
Department of Surgery, Gachon University Gil Hospital, Gachon University of Medicine and Science, Incheon, Korea
e-mail: seongmin_kim@gilhospital.com

S.H. Choi, K. Kasama (eds.), *Bariatric and Metabolic Surgery*,
DOI 10.1007/978-3-642-35591-2_8, © Springer-Verlag Berlin Heidelberg 2014

Fig. 8.1 BMI criteria for Bariatric and Gastrointestinal Metabolic surgery for the Asian Population (From Lakdawala and Bhasker [3])

Recommendations

1. Bariatric/gastrointestinal metabolic surgery should be considered as a treatment option for obesity in people with Asian ethnicity with BMI more than 35 kg/m^2 with or without comorbidities.
2. Bariatric/gastrointestinal metabolic surgery should be considered as a treatment option for obesity in people with Asian ethnicity above a BMI of 32 kg/m^2 with comorbidities.
3. Bariatric/gastrointestinal metabolic surgery should be considered as a treatment option for obesity in people with Asian ethnicity above a BMI of 30 kg/m^2 if they have central obesity (waist circumference more than 80 cm in females and more than 90 cm in males) along with at least two of the additional criteria for metabolic syndrome: raised triglycerides, reduced HDL cholesterol levels, high blood pressure and raised fasting plasma glucose levels.
4. Any surgery done on diabetic patients with a BMI less than 30 kg/m^2 should be strictly done only under study protocol with an informed consent from the patient. The nature of these surgeries should be considered as yet purely experimental only as part of research projects with prior approval of the ethics committee.

In our clinical experience, the ideal LAGB candidate includes relatively young (age <40) and well-motivated patients, female, BMI <50 kg/m^2, and simple obesity without serious comorbidities.

8.3 Pre-op Evaluation wwand Preparation

Proper preoperative patient education is essential and attendance at educational sessions is mandatory. Poor understanding of the concept of food restriction in AGB can be a potential risk factor for post-op complications. We routinely check chest PA, EKG, CBC, serum biochemistry, urinalysis, coagulation profiles, thyroid function test, HbA1C, and lipid profiles (TG, cholesterol, HDL, and LDL). Cholelithiasis or steatohepatitis are the most prevalent of the several gastrointestinal conditions in morbidly obese patients. Abdominal ultrasound is performed for evaluating the gall bladder and liver for patients showing relevant symptoms or elevated liver enzymes. Gynecologic specialist checks the ovary and uterine diseases if there are menstruation-associated problems. Patients with a history of recent chest pain or a change in exercise tolerance need to undergo a formal cardiology assessment, including stress testing and echocardiogram as indicated. Patients with suggestive histories of clinically significant sleep apnea need to undergo preoperative sleep study testing. If found to have the condition, use of a continuous or bi-level positive airway pressure apparatus postoperatively while sleeping can eliminate the stressful periods of hypoxia. Gastroesophageal reflux disease (GERD) is common in severely obese patients because of the increased abdominal pressure and shortened lower esophageal sphincter. Gastrofibroscope is not routinely performed before LAGB, but we performed that for patients who have not undergone an endoscopy before, have GI symptom such as reflux, have epigastralgia, have antireflux medications, and have familial history of esophagogastric malignancy.

The size of the left lobe of the liver often inhibits the surgeon's ability to complete LAGB. Patients with a known enlarged fatty liver may benefit from hypocaloric diet tried for several weeks before surgery for shrinkage of the left lobe of the liver. This facilitates the LAGB procedure without complications such as inaccessibility of the cardiac region or liver capsular bleeding. Preoperatively, SC injections of heparin or low-molecular-weight heparin (LMWH) for DVT prophylaxis is not routinely performed except for those who are high-risk thrombophilic patients including superobese patients anticipating longer procedure, those with history of DVT, venous stasis ulcer, and hypoventilation syndrome of obesity. Recent data have shown that pulmonary embolism is uncommon after laparoscopic bariatric surgery and that measures such as early ambulation and sequential compression devices(SCD), without pharmacologic agents, such as heparin, can be used successfully to prevent DVT and PE in many patients undergoing LAGB [4]. We routinely use perioperative SCD and encourage patients' early ambulation after LAGB. A prophylactic intravenous first-generation cephalosporin, in a dose appropriate for weight, is given preoperatively and, if deemed necessary, intraoperatively (long procedure or contamination). Antibiotics are continued for less than 24 h. Oral antibiotics are prescribed several days as discharge medications with narcotics, antacids, and prokinctics.

8.4 Operation

After induction anesthesia, patients' prep is very important for safely and easily performing the procedure. Urinary catheterization is seldom necessary except in case of difficult case of revisional surgery or complication surgery in which expected procedure time is longer than 2–3 h. Nasogastric tube is not necessary except in case of significant gastric distension after induction anesthesia. Before skin prep of the patients, we always test the mobility of operation table whether or not the steep reverse Trendelenburg position is possible. For most morbidly obese patients, the huge fatty omentum prevents adequate view of the GE junction. Therefore, reverse Trendelenburg position is important for easily accessing the cardia in these patients. Vertical foot plate fixed in the table is very useful for maintenance of the steep reverse Trendelenburg position in this circumstance. The skin is soaped with skin soap. Skin prep with Betadine ranges from upper limit nipple level to lower limit anterior superior iliac spine level. Laterally, margin of surgical prep is slightly lateral to both anterior axillary lines. Antimicrobial Ioban™ incise drape is preferred by some surgeons. We have found a 10 mm/30° telescope, extra-long, atraumatic graspers, and other instruments to be most useful. Extra-long trocars may be needed for superobese patients. An ultrasonic scalpel is helpful in all aspects of the dissection even in AGB procedure. A fixed retractor device secured to the operating room table for clamping and holding the liver retractor is also essential. The surgeon stands to the patient's right, the assistant is to the patient's left, and the camera operator is adjacent to the surgeon.

The standard trocar placement for AGB we usually perform is as follows (Fig. 8.2): The first trocar used is 15 mm trocar at or just above the umbilicus. We usually do this with open Hasson techniques. After CO_2 insufflation until 15 mmHg and under the direct view from the umbilical trocar, additional four trocars are inserted: two 5 mm trocars at both subcostal areas, one 12 mm trocar at left upper quadrant, and 5 mm epigastric trocars for Nathanson liver retractor. For the superobese (e.g., BMI >60), three abdominal trocars need to be moved slightly cephalad direction for better surgical view of cardiac region. Pneumoperitoneum usually ranged within 12–15 mmHg. In case of superobese patients, adjustment up to 20 mmHg level is often necessary for elevating thick abdominal wall. Communication with the anesthesiologist for

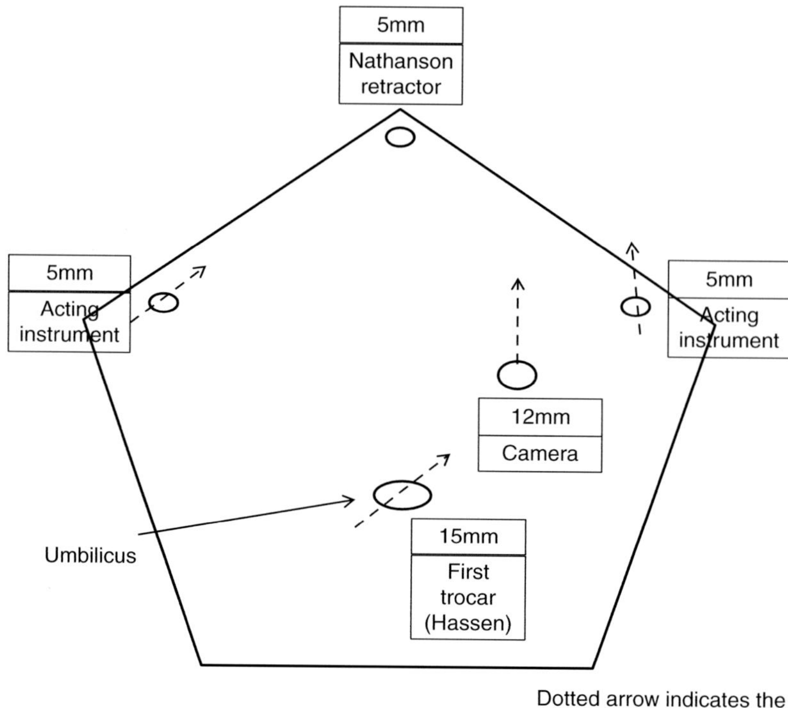

Fig. 8.2 The standard trocar placement for AGB. *Dotted arrow* indicates the direction of trocar advance

adjusting the pressure of air insufflations is very important for preventing CO_2 retention or hypoxia induced by excessive pressure from abdominal cavity.

All operations are performed by the author utilizing LAP-BAND® (Allergan, Irvine, CA, USA) with different modifications (9.75/10.0, AP series). However, the AGB procedure may be performed with any of various types of adjustable bands. They all work on the principle of reduction of oral intake by augmenting the early satiety and decrease in appetite triggered by distention of the proximal part of the stomach. The two bands approved for use by the FDA in the United States are the LAP-BAND® (Allergan, Irvine, CA, USA) and the Realize Band (Ethicon Endo-Surgery, Cincinnati, Ohio). The Swedish Adjustable Gastric Band (Obtech Medical, Baar, Switzerland), the MIDBAND (Medical Innovation Development, Villeurbanne, France), and the Heliogast band (Helioscopie, Vienne, France) are other banding systems used in Europe, Asia, the Middle East, and South America. Key points of the techniques of placement of the AGB include (1) very small pouch formation by placement of the band on top of the stomach just below the gastroesophageal junction. A calibration tube with a 25 cc balloon may be used depending on surgeon's preference for proper band placement and detection of the hiatal defect. (2) The pars flaccida technique, in which entry into the lesser sac is avoided by placement of the band suprabursally around gastric vessels and fat instead of close to the gastric wall. (3) Anterior fixation of the gastric fundus using three to four nonabsorbable sutures between above and below the band.

After adequate liver retraction with Nathanson retractor, access to the gastroesophageal junction becomes much easier. The telescope is placed through the left upper quadrant 12 mm port for this part of the operation to maximally view the angle of His area. Fundus is grasped with babcock forceps and retracted downward to the patient's right side for stretching that area. With a hook diathermy, peritoneal membranes on the phrenoesophageal fat pad at the angle of His are minimally dissected to create an opening in the peritoneum (Fig. 8.3a). Swabbing with suction device in that area is useful for clearly exposing the His angle and left pillar of the crus muscle (Fig. 8.3b). The pars flaccida technique has become the approach of choice for placing the adjustable band. The filmy membranous gastro-hepatic ligament onto the caudate lobe (pars flaccida) is divided for accessing the right pillar of the crus muscle of the diaphragm (Fig. 8.3c). The anterior branch of the vagus nerve and any aberrant left hepatic artery should be preserved at this point of time. Caudate lobe and crus muscle should be seen clearly because occasionally the vena cava can lie close to the caudate lobe. With an ultrasonic device (or hook diathermy), the peritoneal membrane above the right pillar of the crus muscle fascia is minimally dissected and advanced about 1–2 cm toward the patient's left with a gentle spreading and pushing technique (Fig. 8.3d). With laparoscopic grasper, omentum encasing the perigastric vessels is carefully grasped away to the left of the patient. This facilitates band passer entry into the band tunnel opening. Special tunneling instrument (band passer), which follows the surface of the

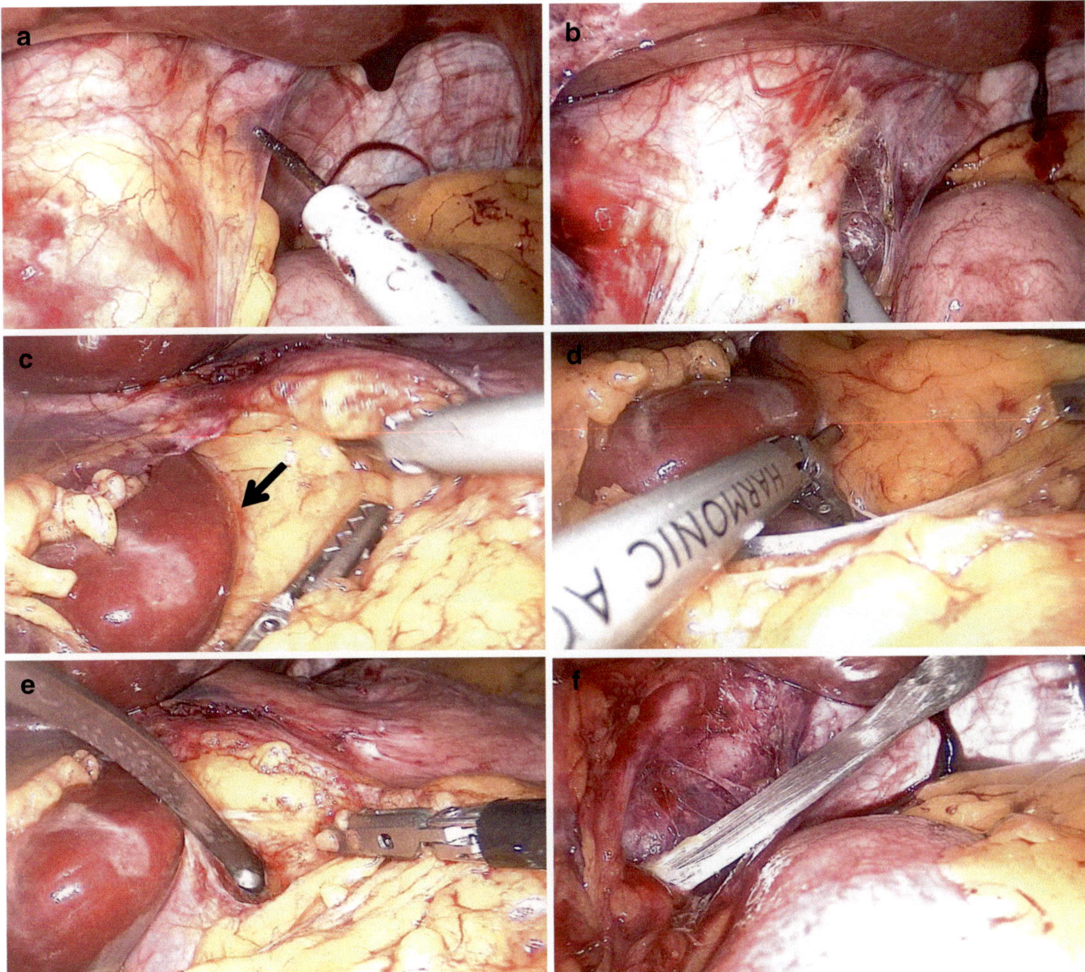

Fig. 8.3 (**a**) Create an opening in the peritoneum. (**b**) Expose the His angle and left pillar of the crus muscle. (**c**) Divide the membranous gastrohepatic ligament. *Arrow* indicates landmark area for starting retrogastric tunneling (between crus muscle and perigastric fat). (**d**) Dissect minimally the peritoneal membrane above the right pillar of the crus muscle fascia. (**e**, **f**) Insert the Band passer smoothly on the surface of the right crus posterior and inferior to the esophagus

right crus posterior and inferior to the esophagus while aiming for the angle of His, should be advanced smoothly without any resistance until it can be seen at the other side near the top of the spleen (Fig. 8.3e, f). Resistance often can be felt during advancement of the band passer in case where the retrogastric tunnel is made incorrectly, for example, (1) below the right crus muscle fascia (2) penetrating the left crus fascia (3) entering the bursa omentalis (lesser sac). In these circumstances, the band passer should be withdrawn and it should be advanced with direct vision carefully. Small blood vessels can bleed, but it usually stops spontaneously or is easily controlled with coagulation. The adjustable band is placed through the large 15 mm trocar. With the guidance of the band passer, the band tubing is introduced into the posterior tunnel and pulled through from the greater to the lesser side of the

stomach. The band is locked using the atraumatic forceps. A 5-mm grasper inserted between the band and stomach ensures that the band is not too tight. Three or four gastrogastric plications over the band with 2-0 nonabsorbable suture material are performed. The first stitch should be located as far posterolateral on fundus as possible because this region has been the most frequent area of fundus herniation through the band. Suture should not be performed in front of the band buckle. The accurate seromuscular bites are very important because inaccurate gastrogastric sutures can be loosened with time and eventually make the portion of the fundus redundant below the band, which is the culprit of the partial fundal prolapse causing anterolateral band slippage. Removal of the fat pad on the cardia with coagulation greatly facilitates the accurate seromuscular bites (Fig. 8.4). Adequate

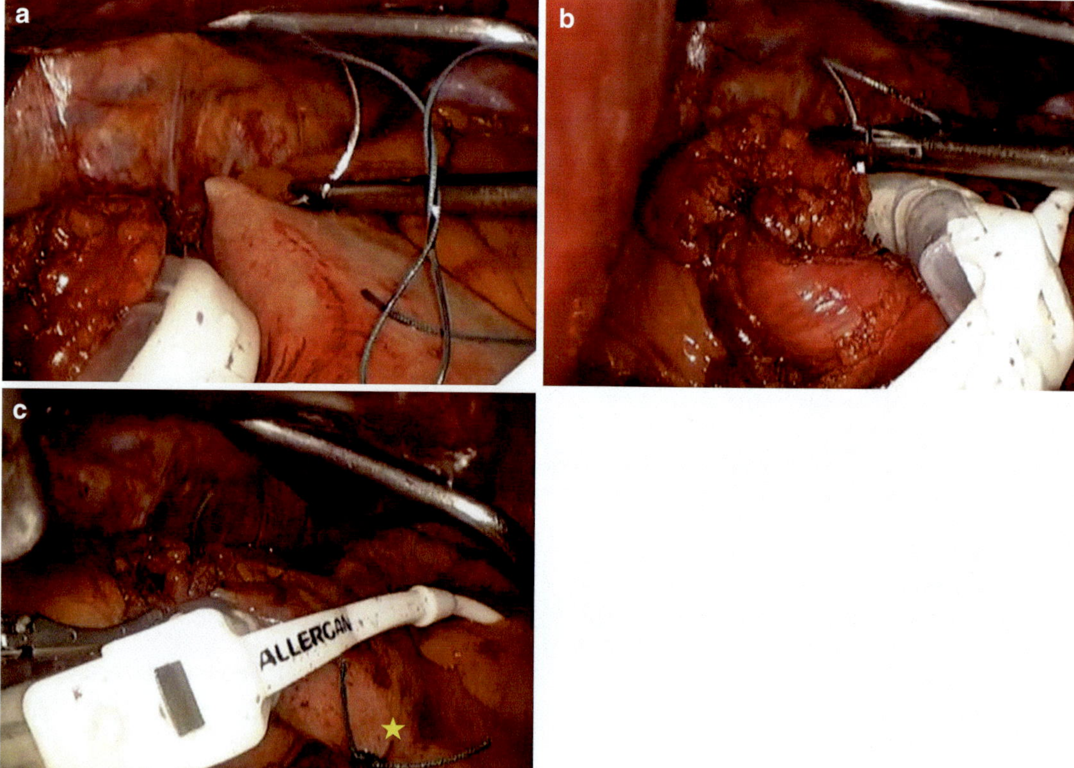

Fig. 8.4 Technical pearls for preventing fundal herniation. (**a**) The first stitch should be located as far posterolateral on fundus as possible. (**b**) Scoring of the thick fat pad on the cardia greatly facilitates the accurate seromuscular bites. (**c**) Anterolateral plication: optional (*star*)

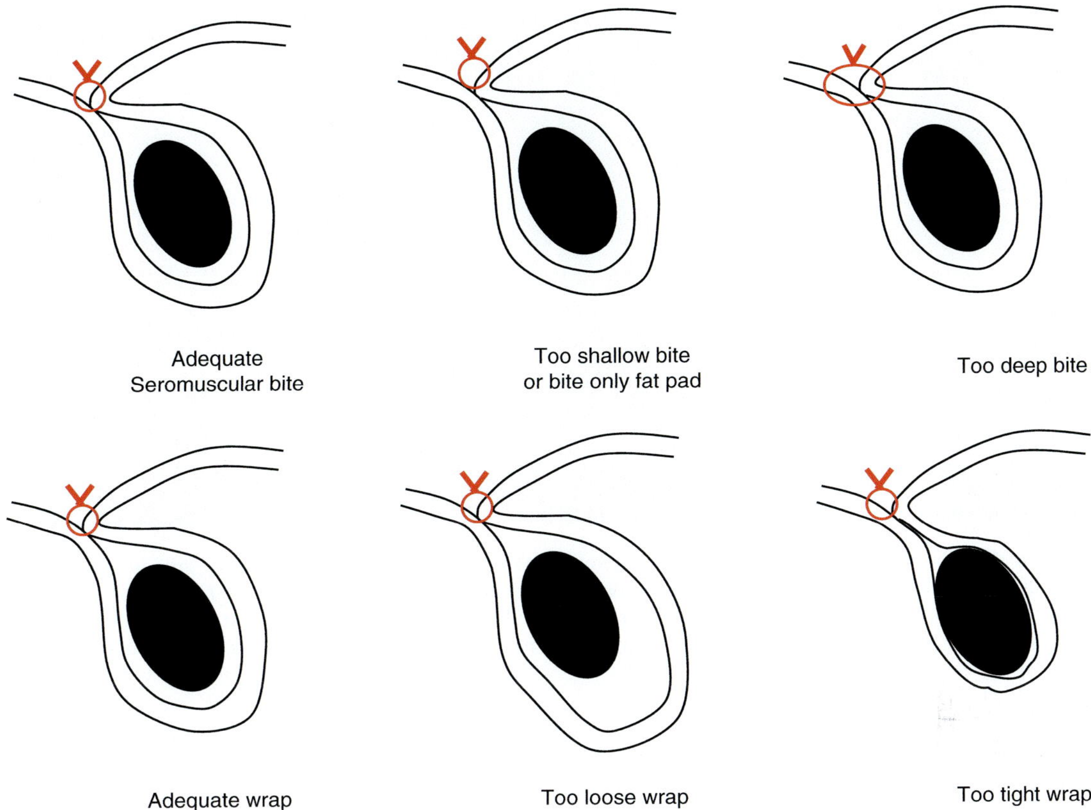

Fig. 8.5 Several types of seromuscular bite and wrap

seromuscular bite and wrap stabilize the gastric band and minimize the complications such as fundal prolapse (slippage) or band erosion (Fig. 8.5). After the intra-abdominal procedure is completed, the tubing is retrieved through one of the trocar sites (usually left upper quadrant). With the laparoscopic grasper inserted through the 15-mm trocar incision site, a subcutaneous tunnel is made, through which the end of the tubing is grasped. The tubing is retrieved through the subcutaneous tunnel, excess tubing is trimmed, and then the port is connected to the tubing. The port is secured onto the anterior rectus fascia by four stitches made with Prolene sutures (Ethicon).

After operation, and returning to ward, we usually keep the patients NPO for 4 h, then encourage mineral water and clear liquid diet sequentially. Adequate pain control is essential. Narcotic requirements are decreased with a laparoscopic approach. A patient-controlled analgesia (PCA) pump is appropriate and helpful. When the patients are deemed to be able to drink total 2 l of water per day, tolerate post-op pain with oral analgesics, and are mobile, they are discharged on the same day or post-op day 1. We do not routinely obtain a radiographic study of the gastrointestinal tract after AGB unless there are clinical signs of a gastric perforation (which include a temperature higher than 100 °C or a heart rate higher than 100 beats/min) or stoma obstruction (sustained vomiting).

8.5 Outpatient Care, Education, and Band Adjustment

Although the schedule of postoperative visits varies, all patients must undergo a long-term follow-up. We usually stitch out tenth post-op day. Diet schedules include 2 weeks of liquid diet, then 2 weeks of soft diet. We encourage patients

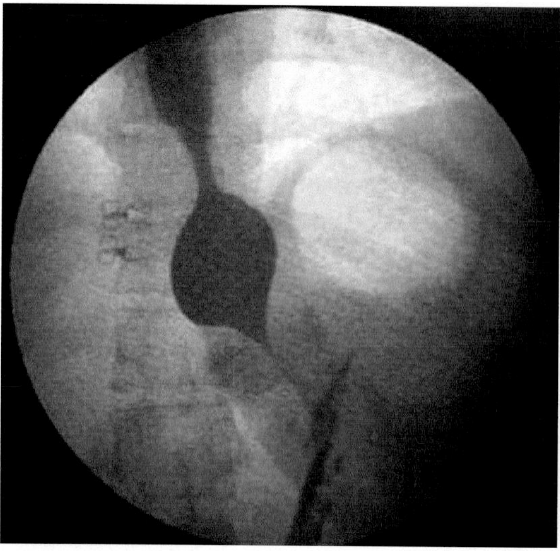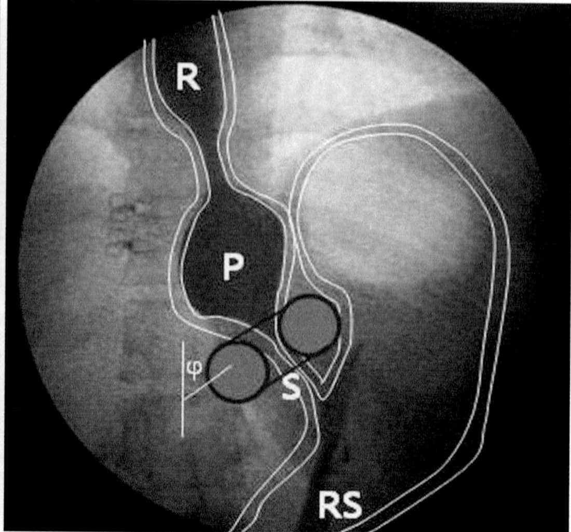

Fig. 8.6 Patterns of normal barium passage in fluoroscopy-guided band adjustment. Following addition of saline in the band, swallowed barium is suspended, resulting in temporary formation of a small pouch (*P*) above the band. Within several seconds, barium passes through the narrow stoma (*S*), which should be grossly equal to the width of the tubing (approximately 4 mm). Temporary mild reflux (*R*) of barium is noted. All swallowed barium passes through the band by the secondary esophageal contraction within 10–15 s. *RS* remnant stomach

to try regular diet after post-op 1 month. We emphasize very intensively the need for eating slowly with small bites and chewing well for minimizing food trouble in the patients fitted with gastric band. Improved weight loss occurs in patients who see their surgeon for adjustments to the band. A goal of 0.5–1 kg/week of weight loss is adjusted for initial body weight. We do not perform intraoperative band filling. The band system is left empty with the cuff deflated following surgery. We do the first band adjustment on the 6th post-op week. We have adopted fluoroscopy-guided band adjustment. However, it can be performed in the office or clinic without fluoroscopic guidance depending on preference of the clinician. In our adjustment protocol, elective band adjustment is usually performed three times at 1 month interval. After each adjustment, we check the barium swallow passage. We consider several points of fluoroscopic appearance of barium passage as "adequate" adjustment (e.g., stoma diameter of 3–4 mm, transient barium reflux, and complete barium passage through the stoma with several secondary esophageal contractions) (Fig. 8.6). After three elective band adjustments, we do minor band adjustment

(± 0.3 cc) without barium swallow depending on the patient's request regarding regular weight loss, hunger, and meal size. Blood tests after LAGB are seldom performed periodically throughout the patient's follow-up unless there are metabolic indications, patient's underlying medical illnesses, and other indications.

8.6 Outpatient Complications After LAGB

8.6.1 Stoma Obstruction

Not infrequently, patients visit outpatient clinic with symptoms of stoma obstruction during aftercare. Probably, food stuck with poor eating habit (eating too rapidly or not chewing well, too bigger bite) or excessive band adjustment (too tight band) are two common causes of stoma obstruction. Patients should be educated to keep NPO for significant period of time, then sips of warm and clear water whenever there are stuck symptoms. In case of sustained vomiting, band adjustment (remove saline) should be performed immediately, whereas those who show sustained vomiting immediately after LAGB implies misplacement of band or band malfunction; therefore, in these circumstances, the cause of the symptom should be sought actively (with fluoroscopy or endoscopy). Sustained vomiting can cause esophagitis, Mallory-Weiss tear, and gastric prolapse.

8.6.2 Heartburn/Transient Reflux

More commonly, these symptoms are caused by too tight band or poor eating habit of the patients. Small removal of saline from the band is usually effective for alleviating these symptoms. Short course of PPI antacid plus prokinetics use after band deflation are also helpful. Those who complain new-onset reflux symptoms may have slipped gastric band. Therefore, these patients should be checked for band system configuration with fluoroscopy.

8.6.3 Pouch Dilatation/Gastric Prolapse with Band Slippage

For particular symptoms, such as vomiting, reflux, and abdominal pain, we also perform a barium swallow study during the adjustment. Band slippage may result in failed weight loss and/or acute obstruction of the stoma. The frequency depends on patient compliance, surgical technique, and postoperative care, and also may be decreased with patient training to encourage appropriate eating behaviors. Overeating with overfilling of the gastric pouch, overinflation of the gastric band at the time of adjustments, and excessive vomiting are risk factors for band slippage [5]. Pouch dilatation is classified as concentric and eccentric. Eccentric pouch dilatation is always accompanied by band slippage, which is classified as anterior and postoperative slippage. Therefore, complications of pouch dilatation with/without band slippage are codified as follows: CP, concentric pouch dilatation (normal band angle) (Fig. 8.7); EPA1, eccentric pouch with early anterior slippage (normal band angle with a ringlike configuration); EPA2, eccentric

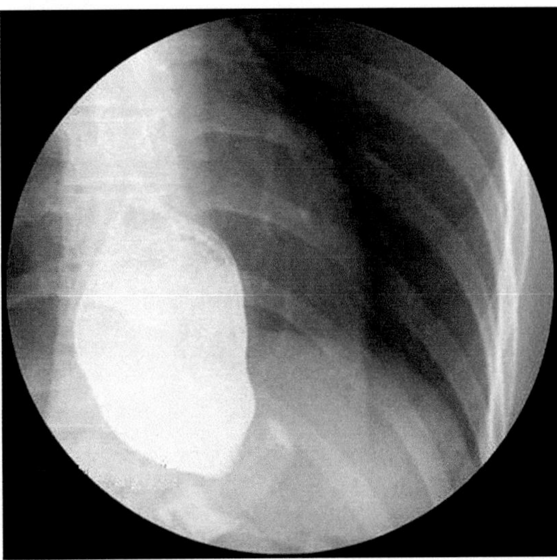

Fig. 8.7 Concentric pouch dilatation (CP). Normal band position and normal band angle are noted. The pouch is dilated concentrically. The pouch appears to have migrated to the intrathoracic level, suggesting the presence of a coexisting hiatal hernia

pouch with chronic anterior slippage (a more horizontal band angle); EPA3, eccentric pouch with acute anterior slippage (an overwhelming pouch covers the band or clockwise rotation of the band with downward migration); and EPP, eccentric pouch with posterior slippage (the band was noted as having counterclockwise rotation with a huge air-fluid pocket inferior and posterior of the band) (Fig. 8.8). Conservative treatment includes total or near-total removal of saline in the band and gradual readjustment with great care for recurrence of abnormal clinico-radiologic signs and symptoms. Strict dietary education is also administered during the "rest" period. Readjustment is usually started around 3–4 weeks after total removal of saline. For patients who do not respond to the conservative management, surgical treatment (repositioning or replacing the band) should be considered.

8.6.4 Band Erosion

Intragastric erosion, penetration, or migration of the band is a major long-term complication following LAGB. Band erosion (BE) requires

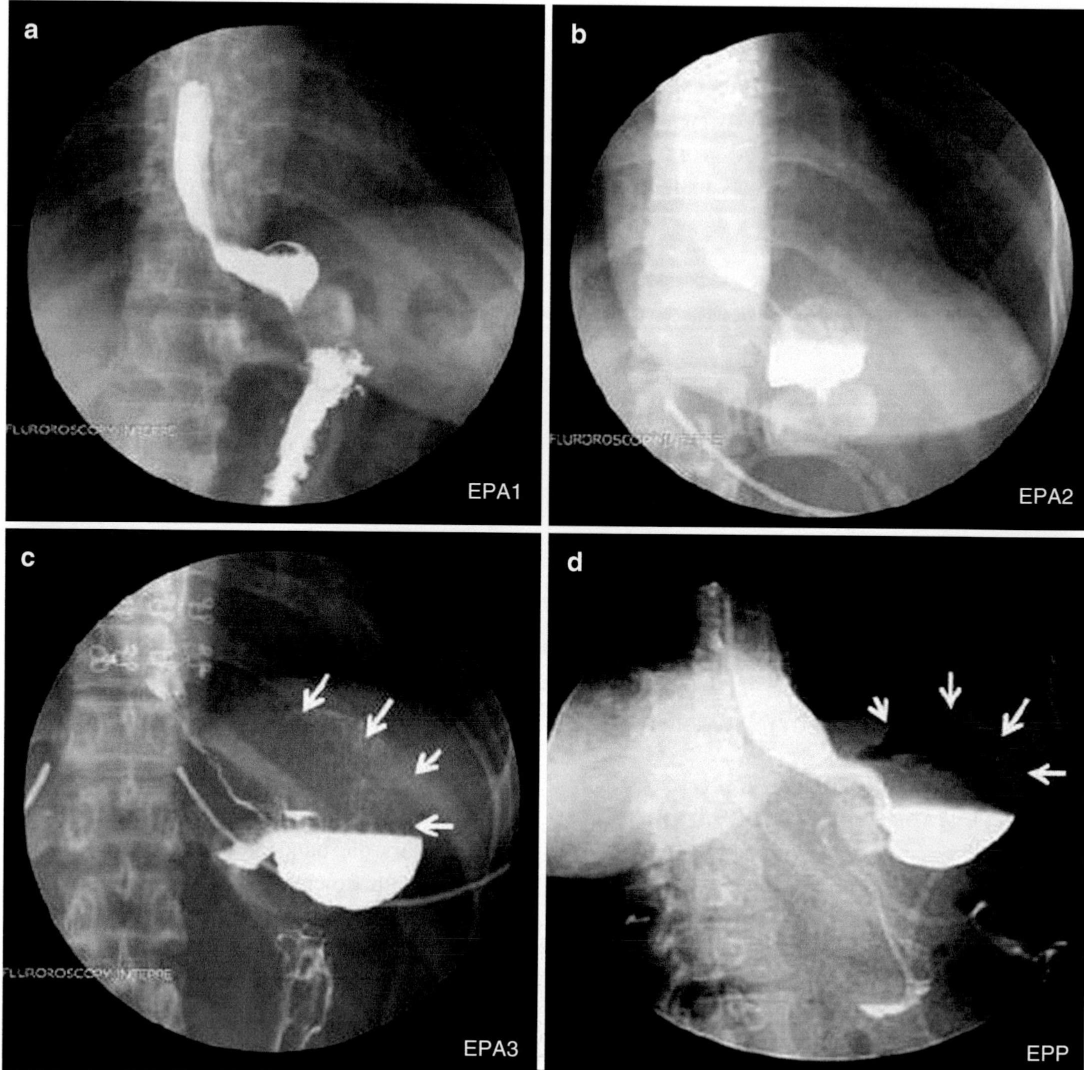

Fig. 8.8 Upper GI study of eccentric pouch dilatation. (**a**) EPA1, eccentric pouch with a normal band angle with a ring-like band configuration. Radiologically, this type is early anterior slippage. (**b**) EPA2, eccentric pouch with a more horizontal band angle. This type of dilatation usually results in a progressive chronic symptom of acid reflux. (**c**) EPA3, eccentric pouch with excessive clockwise rotation of the band. This type of dilatation usually manifests as acute, total food intolerance with severe reflux and epigastric pain. (**d**) EPP, eccentric pouch with posterior band slippage. This type of dilatation is associated with use of poor surgical techniques (e.g., entering the lesser sac with a redundant posterior gastric wall). *Arrows* indicates outlines for prolapsed gastric pouch above the band

removal of the gastric band system. With this complication, the gastric band gradually erodes or migrates into the gastric wall. According to the literature, BE after LAGB in high-volume center occurs in about 0.23–8.94 % of cases [6, 7]. There is neither clear-cut symptom nor exact etiopathology of the BE [7]. We speculate "microtrauma" of the pouch as the culprit of BE (e.g., intraoperative damage, NSAID, excessive vomiting, overinflation of the band, band infection). Asymptomatic individuals can often increase their food intake and gain weight. However, in our series of patients, nonspecific abdominal pain was the predominant symptom, which is in line with findings from other studies. 83 % complained of upper abdominal pain, and port infection was present in 50 %. On rare occasion, patients presented with acute peritonitis or nonemergent GI bleeding. Based on the clinical signs and symptoms suggestive of BE, upper gastrointestinal (UGI) and abdominal CT scan are helpful. The barium swallow test typically shows barium passing from the upper to the lower gastric pouch outside the band. Abdominal CT scan can detect small free air or localized abscess formation around the band, tube, and reservoir port. EGD is the definitive study instrument of choice.

On EGD, the band typically protrudes into the gastric lumen. Occasionally, pus (infected purulent fluid) descending down from the pouch near the GE junction may be the only sign of BE on retroversion at endoscopy (Fig. 8.9). There is no consensus on the technique of removal of the eroded gastric band. In our series of patients, all eroded bands were removed via direct dissection outside the stomach because we decided that the band was easily identified along the connecting tube following dissection. However, the fibrous capsule around the band is actually "unhealthy" phlegmonous tissue. Therefore, after removal of

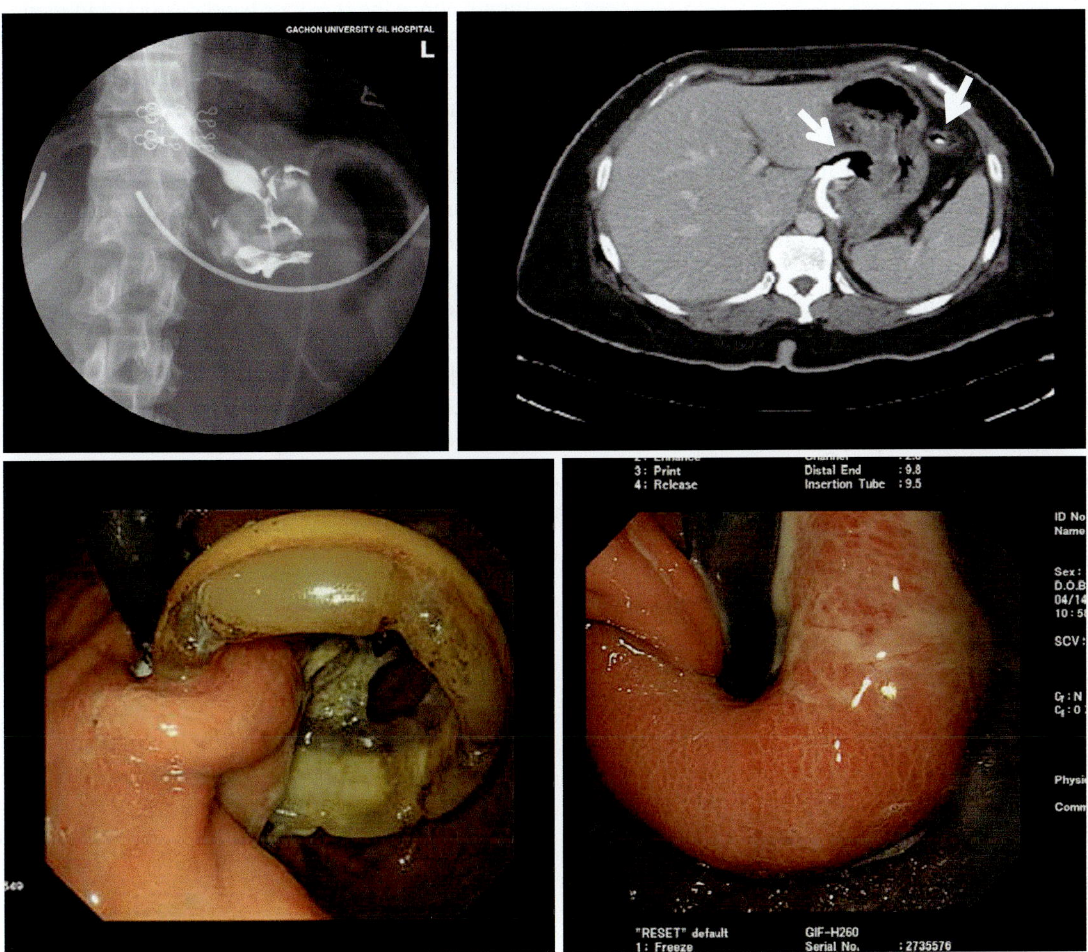

Fig. 8.9 Band erosion. The barium swallow test shows barium passing from the upper to the lower gastric pouch outside the band. Abdominal CT scan detects small free air and localized abscess formation around the band. On EGD, the band protrudes into the gastric lumen. Pus (infected purulent fluid) descending down from the pouch near the GE junction is shown

the band, closure of the remaining gastric perforation is very difficult, and repaired gastrostomies are more prone to leakage and breakdown. Recent reports also suggest that endoscopic removal of the eroded band is a feasible procedure [8, 9]. Endoscopic removal of an eroded band may require multiple sessions, and patient symptoms might prevent postponement of the procedure while waiting for the erosion to progress. However, we prefer endoscopic removal of eroded gastric band because it is a nonoperative option and therefore avoids surgery and general anesthesia. Minimal scar tissue after endoscopic removal facilitates future secondary bariatric procedure [8].

8.6.5 Port-Related Problems

Unlike the well-known complications such as slippage, erosion, and infection, port complications are still underestimated because they have been considered minor problems, and relatively few require surgical treatment. The port, however, is the Achilles' heel of gastric band surgery, and access-port complications are actually the most frequent complication. According to the literatures, as many as 4–20 % of patients have port complications [10, 11], which include infection, inversion/migration that makes accessing port impossible, associated skin erosion, abdominal wall hernia, and leakage of saline. Port-related problems may be unavoidable because both the port and the tubing are subject to wear and tear. However, most of the port problem can be corrected under local anesthesia (port removal and/or exchange). Port infection remote from surgery should be regarded as a sign of band erosion and needs endoscopic examination because presumably the infection from eroded band tracks down via the tubing to the port.

8.7 Revisional Surgery

Revisional surgery or secondary gastric banding (rebanding) are often necessary for LAGB complications. We summarize the technical aspects of LAGB revision in two common situations: slippage and erosion. Except urgent band removal in case of an acute stoma obstruction with excessively large or partially necrotic gastric pouch, the ideal revisional surgery for slipped gastric band is removal and repositioning because recurrent slippage is prone to occur after the simple reduction of prolapse and resuturing [12]. Removal and repositioning procedure consists of repositioning of the gastric band through the newly formed retrogastric tunnel above the previous band position and meticulous fixation sutures of redundant gastric pouch around the band. If hiatal hernia is grossly evident, it requires concurrent repair (Fig. 8.10). Rebanding after band erosion is often requested by the patient because of significant regain of body weight after band removal. However, if the patient is not pleased with the first band, a different bariatric operation should be considered. The outcome of the rebanding after band erosion has been disappointing because of unacceptably high incidence of re-erosion [8]. However, for those whose band had been removed during early stage of erosion or removed by endoscopy, rebanding can be performed without difficulty. It can be performed at least 3 months after band removal. Retrogastric tunneling slightly above the previous band position should be performed because dissection of scar near the previous band position is very difficult or not possible at all. Careful dissection and advancement under the crus muscle fascia (subfascial approach) minimizes the chance of gastric perforation during the rebanding procedure (Fig. 8.11). Endoscopic examination is recommended after the procedure before awaking the patient if there is a concern for gastric perforation.

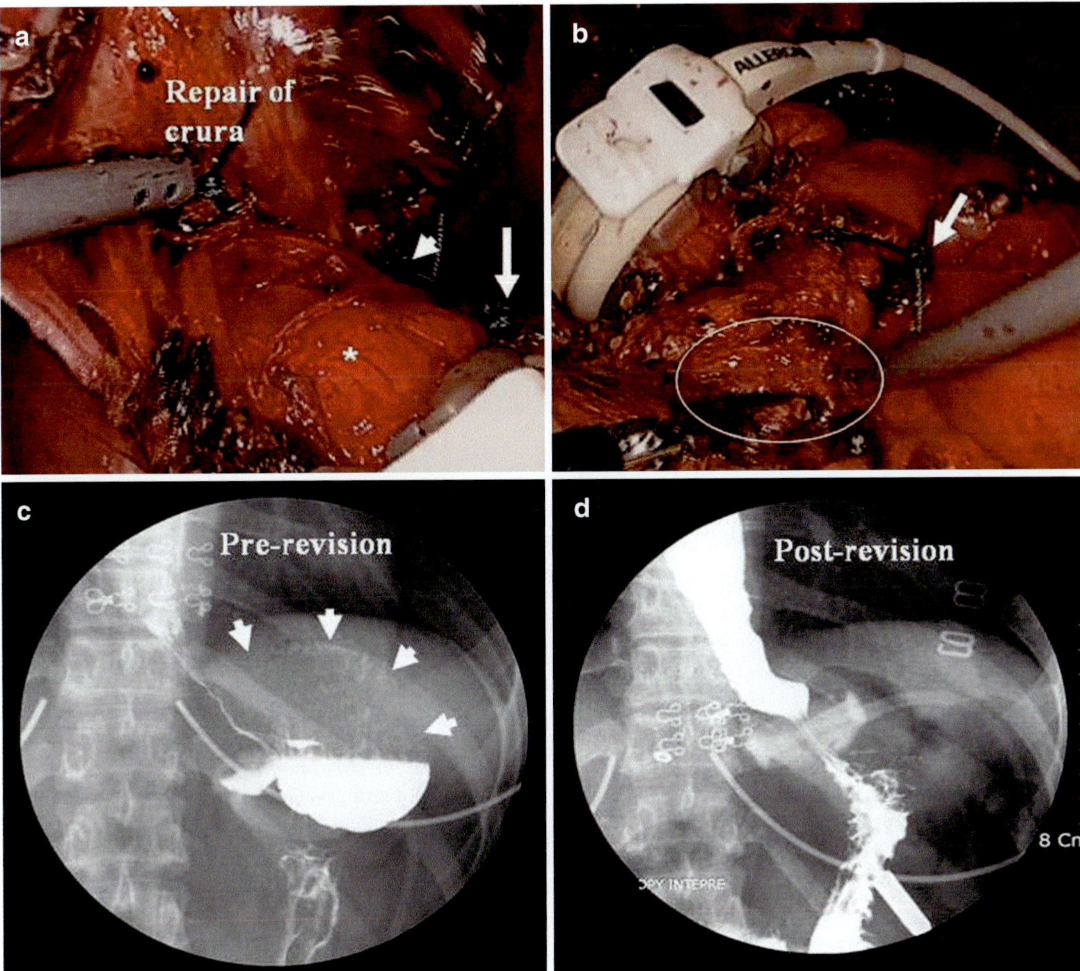

Fig. 8.10 Laparoscopic nondestructive removal of the band and its repositioning at a proper level in an EPA3 patient. (**a**) In patients with pouch enlargement with severe reflux, a variable degree of hiatal hernia was usually observed, and we performed concomitant repair using figure of eight sutures of the anterior crura muscle. Plicated neofundus was anchored to the crural muscle fascia (*short arrow*), and gastrogastric suture was also performed (*long arrow*). *Asterisk*: newly formed pouch. (**b**) Repositioning of the gastric band through the newly formed retrogastric tunnel above the previous band position (*circular area*). Anterior plication of the gastric wall below the band was performed (*arrow*). Pre-op (**c**) and post-op (**d**) Gastrografin swallow study showed that the band angle and pouch shape (*arrow*) were normalized

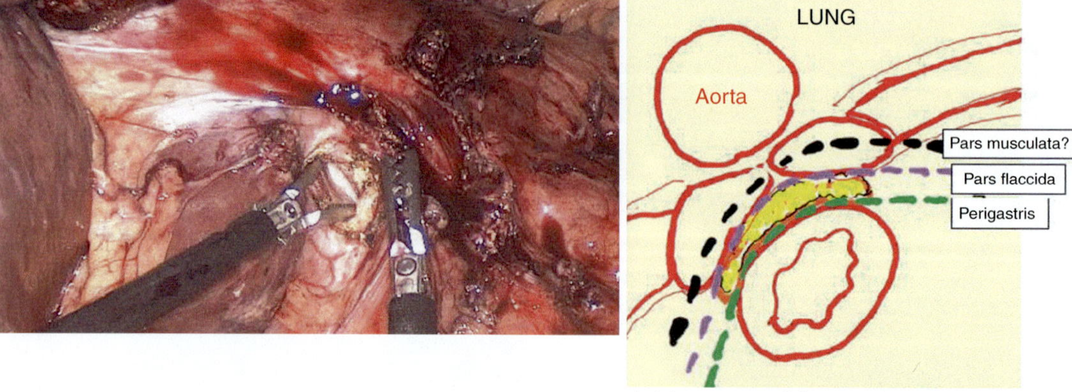

Axial anatomy of the esophageal hiatus

Fig. 8.11 Repositioning of the gastric band through the newly formed retrogastric tunnel above the previous band position (subfascial approach)

Further Videos

Electronic supplementary material is available in the online version of this chapter at (doi:10.1007/978-3-642-35591-2_8) and accessible for authorised users. Videos can also be accessed at http://www.springerimages.com/videos/978-3-642-35590-5

References

1. Buchwald H, Oien DM. Metabolic/bariatric surgery worldwide 2011. Obes Surg. 2013;23:427–36.
2. O'Brien PE, MacDonald L, Anderson M, Brennan L, Brown WA. Long-term outcomes after bariatric surgery: fifteen-year follow-up of adjustable gastric banding and a systematic review of the bariatric surgical literature. Ann Surg. 2013;257:87–94.
3. Lakdawala M, Bhasker A. Report: Asian Consensus Meeting on Metabolic Surgery. Recommendations for the use of bariatric and gastrointestinal metabolic surgery for treatment of obesity and type II diabetes mellitus in the Asian population: August 9th and 10th, 2008, Trivandrum, India. Obes Surg. 2010;20:929–36.
4. Clements RH, Yellumahanthi K, Ballem N, Wesley M, Bland KI. Pharmacologic prophylaxis against venous thromboembolic complications is not mandatory for all laparoscopic Roux-en-Y gastric bypass procedures. J Am Coll Surg. 2009;208:917–21; discussion 21–3.
5. Carucci LR, Turner MA, Szucs RA. Adjustable laparoscopic gastric banding for morbid obesity: imaging assessment and complications. Radiol Clin North Am. 2007;45:261–74.
6. Nocca D, Frering V, Gallix B, de Seguin des Hons C, Noel P, Foulonge MA, et al. Migration of adjustable gastric banding from a cohort study of 4236 patients. Surg Endosc. 2005;19:947–50.
7. Egberts K, Brown WA, O'Brien PE. Systematic review of erosion after laparoscopic adjustable gastric banding. Obes Surg. 2011;21:1272–9.
8. Chisholm J, Kitan N, Toouli J, Kow L. Gastric band erosion in 63 cases: endoscopic removal and rebanding evaluated. Obes Surg. 2011;21:1676–81.
9. Neto MP, Ramos AC, Campos JM, Murakami AH, Falcao M, Moura EH, et al. Endoscopic removal of eroded adjustable gastric band: lessons learned after 5 years and 78 cases. Surg Obes Relat Dis. 2010;6:423–7.
10. Lyass S, Cunneen SA, Hagiike M, Misra M, Burch M, Khalili TM, et al. Device-related reoperations after laparoscopic adjustable gastric banding. Am Surg. 2005;71:738–43.
11. Lattuada E, Zappa MA, Mozzi E, Antonini I, Boati P, Roviaro GC. Injection port and connecting tube complications after laparoscopic adjustable gastric banding. Obes Surg. 2010;20:410–4.
12. Manganiello M, Sarker S, Tempel M, Shayani V. Management of slipped adjustable gastric bands. Surg Obes Relat Dis. 2008;4:534–8; discussion 38.

Kyung Yul Hur

9.1 Background

The first gastric bypass surgery was performed by Mason and Ito in 1966. They divided stomach horizontally and created a loop gastroenterostomy between proximal gastric pouch and jejunum. However, the proximal gastric pouch in this procedure was high up in the abdomen, close to the gastroesophageal junction. This caused bile reflux and led to esophagitis. In addition, the high location of anastomosis also led to technical difficulties. Also, the transverse pouch led to dilation of fundus and failure of effective weight loss.

The mini-gastric bypass (Fig. 9.1) was developed to overcome these limitations by Rutledge in the 1990s. In the mini-gastric bypass, the gastric tube is made parallel to the lesser curvature and the gastric fundus is excluded from the gastric tube. The anastomosis and the jejuna loop are placed low on the stomach, just proximal to the pyloric ring. In this way, the mini-gastric bypass could have reversibility and simplicity of procedure.

9.2 Procedure

9.2.1 Patient Position

Patients are placed in about 30° reverse Trendelenburg position or supine position with or without legs apart. The operating room table should be able to bear the weight of the patient.

9.2.2 Establish the Pneumoperitoneum

Insert 10-mm trocar for laparoscope entry at or over the umbilicus by open Hasson technique or by a Veress needle technique. 11- or 12-mm trocar with zero-degree scope can be used just below the left subcostal margin. CO_2 insufflation between 14 and 18 mmHg would be adequate to achieve good operative field. Once the pneumoperitoneum has been established, another working trocars can be placed under direct visualization.

9.2.3 Placement of Trocars

Five or six trocars are used: one 10 mm for the laparoscope, three 12 mm for instruments – especially, linear staplers and intestinal clamps – and one or more 5 mm for retractors and first assistant. A local anesthetic agent can be used to infiltrate the neurovascular plane of abdominal wall prior to insert trocars to reduce postoperative trocar site pain.

K.Y. Hur, MD, PhD
Department of Surgery, Soonchunhyang University Hospital, 59, Daesagwan-ro, Yongsan-gu, Seoul 140-743, Republic of Korea
e-mail: hurusa@hanmail.net

S.H. Choi, K. Kasama (eds.), *Bariatric and Metabolic Surgery*,
DOI 10.1007/978-3-642-35591-2_9, © Springer-Verlag Berlin Heidelberg 2014

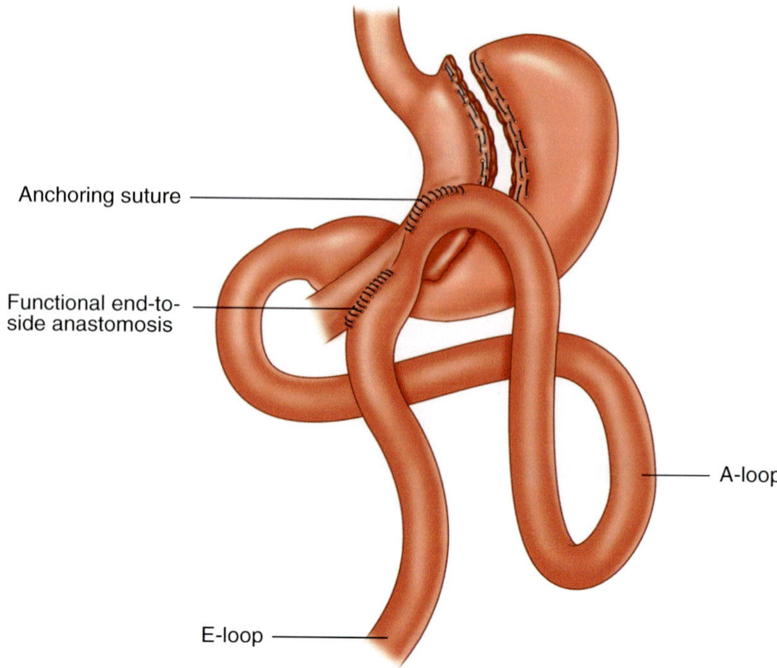

Fig. 9.1 Schematic view of mini-gastric bypass

9.2.4 Retraction of the Liver

Various types of retractor can be used to retract the left hemiliver. Use of a Nathanson, Goldfinger retractors, or use of Endo Peanut as a retractor through an epigastric port (usually 5 mm) might be enough to retract heavy livers; otherwise thread through round ligament and upward retract usually will be sufficient.

9.2.5 Creation of Gastric Pouch and Gastrojejunostomy

A long, narrow gastric tube was created from just proximal to the pyloric ring of lesser curvature toward the angle of His. Then a loop gastroenterostomy was made with the small bowel about 200 cm distal to the ligament of Treitz with linear stapler loaded with tan cartridges (Covidien) or blue cartridges (Ethicon). Entry site of stapler is repaired with continuous suture or another linear stapler. The laparoscopic linear stapler for GI tract anastomosis loaded with purple cartridges (Covidien) or gold cartridges (Ethicon) is used to create the gastric tube.

9.3 Tips

The MGB is a simple, straightforward operation and easy to perform that has low risk and effective in getting and maintaining large amount of weight loss. There is few specific tip needed for this procedure.

However, it is helpful to keep in mind several recommendations:

1. To make the anchoring suture at the midportion of the gastric pouch with the jejunum facilitates parallel line between the pouch and the efferent loop. In this way, the author thinks one can reduce bile refluxes through more physiologic position of the anastomosis and direction of bile flow.
2. To avoid insufficient weight loss or weight regain, it is important not to leave the gastric

pouch large. Surgeons should pay closer attention not to leave redundant posterior wall of the gastric tube for this purpose. Doing countertraction of remnant gastric portion when making gastric tube will help make slender gastric tube.

Further Reading

Buchwald H, Buchwald JN. Evolution of operative procedures for the management of morbid obesity 1950–2000. Obes Surg. 2002;12:819–24.

Rutledge R. The mini-gastric bypass patient and physician resource manual of the Centers for Laparoscopic Obesity Surgery (CLOS). http://clos.net/.

Rutledge R. The mini-gastric bypass: experience with the first 1,274 cases. Obes Surg. 2001;11:276–80.

Rutledge R, Walsh TR. Continued excellent results with the mini-gastric bypass: six-year study in 2,410 patient. Obes Surg. 2005;15:1304–8.

Wang W, Wei PL, Lee YC, Huang MT, Chiu CC, Lee WJ. Short-term results of laparoscopic mini-gastric bypass. Obes Surg. 2005;15:648–54.

Carbajo M, Carcia-Caballero M, Toledano M, Osorio D, Carcia-Lanza C, Carmona JA. One-anastomosis gastric bypass by laparoscopy: results of the first 209 patients. Obes Surg. 2005;15:398–404.

Lee WJ, Yu PJ, Wang W, Chen TC, Wei PL, Huang MT. Laparoscopic Roux-en-Y versus mini-gastric bypass for the treatment of morbid obesity. A prospective randomized controlled clinical trial. Ann Surg. 2005;242:20–8.

Noun R, Skaff J, Riachi E, Daher R, Antoun NA, Nasr M. One thousand consecutive mini-gastric bypass: short- and long-term outcome. Obes Surg. 2012;22:697–703.

Laparoscopic Sleeve Gastrectomy with Duodenal Jejunal Bypass: (LSG/DJB)

Kazunori Kasama

10.1 Introduction

Obesity and metabolic disorders are becoming big issues in Asia. Laparoscopic Roux-en-Y gastric bypass (LRYGB) is still the most popular bariatric procedure in the world. However, in Asia, especially in Korea and Japan, gastric cancer is a common disease, and LRYGB may create an issue related to the bypassed stomach, in regard to the occurrence of a gastric disease as well as carcinoma.

Laparoscopic sleeve gastrectomy (LSG) allows a physiologic passage of food without leaving any gastric segments blind to food and diagnostic study. LSG has been effective for weight loss and reduction of appetite even for Asian people. This is due to the postoperative reduced levels of ghrelin. At the same time, the exclusion of the proximal small intestine from contact with ingested nutrients and faster passage to the distal small intestine could improve glucose tolerance. Combining the advantage of LSG and duodenal jejunal bypass (DJB) may lead to a

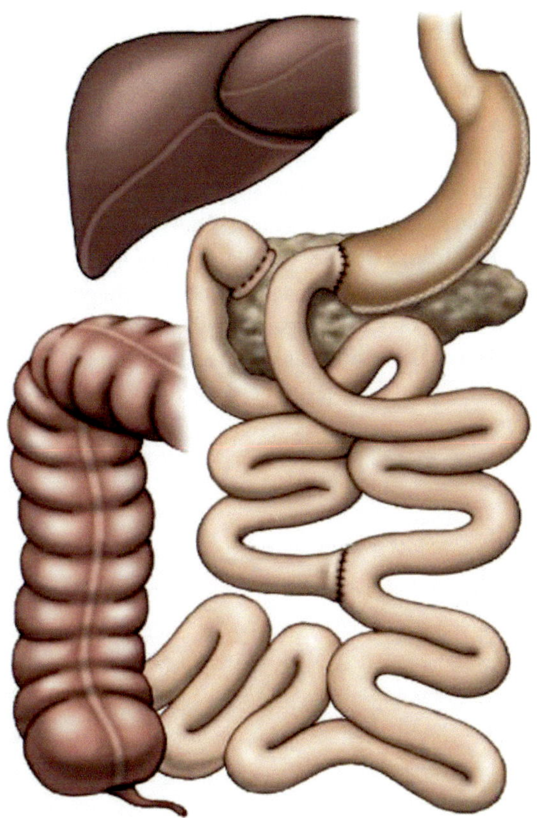

Fig. 10.1 Laparoscopic sleeve gastrectomy (LSG) and duodenal jejunal bypass (DJB)

safer and more effective bariatric procedure (Fig. 10.1) [1].

LSG/DJB may be performed on patients who have fulfilled the bariatric and metabolic surgery indications as well as risk factors of bypassed stomach cancer.

K. Kasama, MD, FACS
Weight Loss and Metabolic Surgery Center,
Yotsuya Medical Cube, 7-7 Nibancho, Chiyoda-ku,
Tokyo 102-0084, Japan
e-mail: kazukasama@gmail.com

S.H. Choi, K. Kasama (eds.), *Bariatric and Metabolic Surgery*,
DOI 10.1007/978-3-642-35591-2_10, © Springer-Verlag Berlin Heidelberg 2014

Risk factors of gastric cancer are determined as follows:

1. *Helicobacter pylori* (*H. pylori*) positive
2. Atrophic change of gastric mucosa, including intestinal metaplasia with or without *H. pylori* infection
3. Family history of gastric cancer

10.2 Operative Technique

The patient should be in the supine position, under general anesthesia, with their legs separated. Five trocars are used as seen in Fig. 10.2. The supra-umbilical trocar is for the camera, and the 5 mm port at the subxyphoid is for the liver retractor. Two 12 mm trocars are placed at the left subcostal margin and 10 cm below that 12 mm trocar. A 15 mm trocar is placed at the upper right abdomen to retrieve the specimen. The position of trocars is the same as when performing LSG.

Regarding the sleeve gastrectomy, the technical aspects are mentioned in another chapter. We will focus on DJB parts in this chapter.

The DJB parts are (1) dissection of the duodenum, (2) jejunojejunostomy, and (3) duodenojejunostomy.

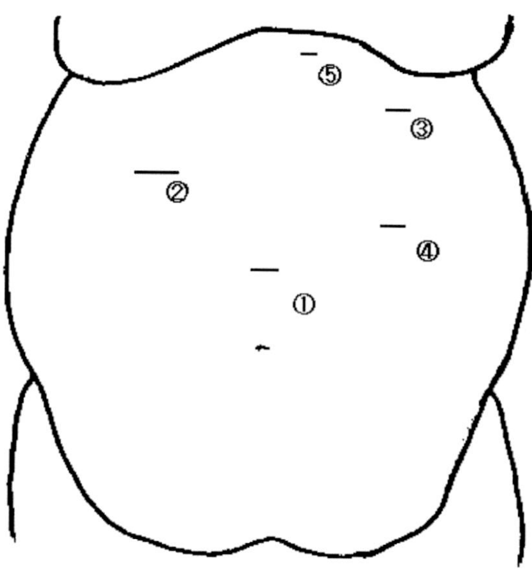

Fig. 10.2 Trocar placement

In this chapter, we would like to show the pictures from an outside view to show the readers the position of the surgeon and how the surgery is performed.

10.2.1 Dissection of Duodenum (Fig. 10.3)

For LSG, devascularization of the gastroepiploic artery is usually started from 4 to 5 cm proximal of the pyloric ring. DJB requires a dissection of the duodenum, so that dissection needs to be continued distally to approximately 1.5 cm beyond the pylorus. Instrument palpation is used to confirm the position of pylorus. The retro-duodenal and supra-duodenal tissues are dissected free in order to facilitate transection of the duodenum at this point with a blue or purple cartridge linear stapler. The right gastric artery should be preserved to maintain the blood supply to the anastomosis. Extra care must be taken during this step because an injury to the pancreas posterior to this point may lead to a lethal complication. The wall of duodenum is thinner than that of the stomach, so the surgeon must make sure to avoid a cavitation injury when using the laparoscopic coagulating shears (LCS).

The transection of the duodenum is performed after LSG is completed (Fig. 10.4). We usually put reticulating linear staples from the left lower trocar to transect the duodenum at a right angle to the duodenum. Usually we use a blue or purple 60 mm stapler. If there is bleeding from the staple line, it is helpful to use sutures.

10.2.2 Jejunojejunostomy

The omentum is displaced cephalad to expose the ligament of Traiz (Fig. 10.5). The omentum of patients undergoing this procedure is heavier than that of patients of average weight, and thus extra care must be taken to avoid injuring the omentum. Placing the omentum beneath the liver keeps it in the best position. The jejunum is transected 100 cm from the ligament of Traiz with a white or camel stapler, and the mesentery is divided with the LCS for 3–4 cm (Fig. 10.6).

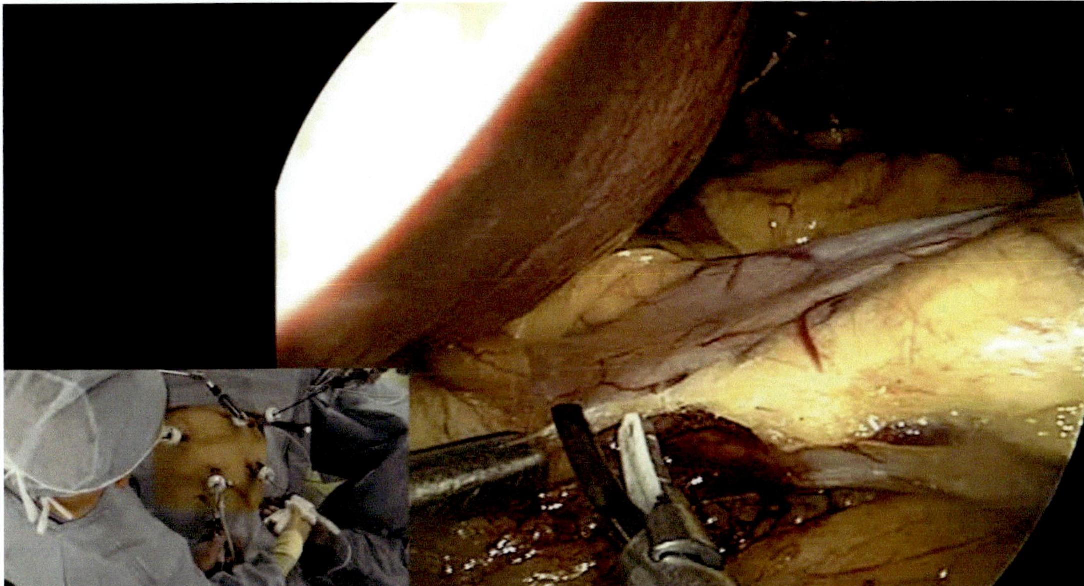

Fig. 10.3 Dissection of the duodenum

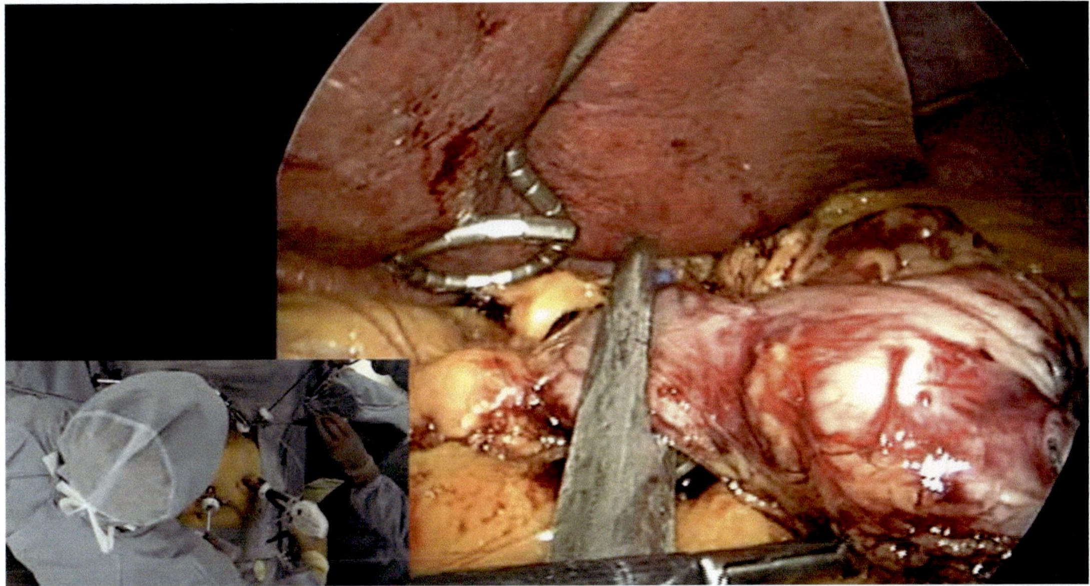

Fig. 10.4 Transection of the duodenum

The assistant should hold the oral side of transected jejunum so it does not get lost while counting the length of the Roux limb, which is usually 150 cm in length.

Two stay sutures are placed at the proximal and distal position of anastomosis in order to fit the axis of anastomosis to that of the stapler. LCS is used to open the entry hole of the stapler (Fig. 10.7), and a white or camel 60 mm linear stapler is inserted through the entry hole to make the jejunojejunostomy (Fig. 10.8). It is necessary to confirm that there is no bleeding from the

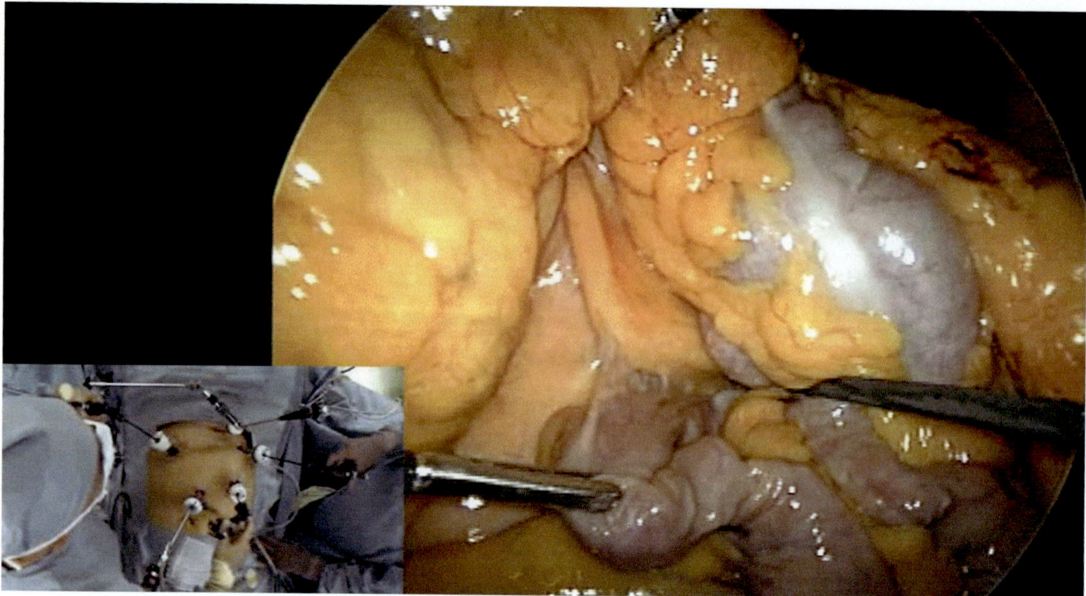

Fig. 10.5 Expose the ligament of Traitz

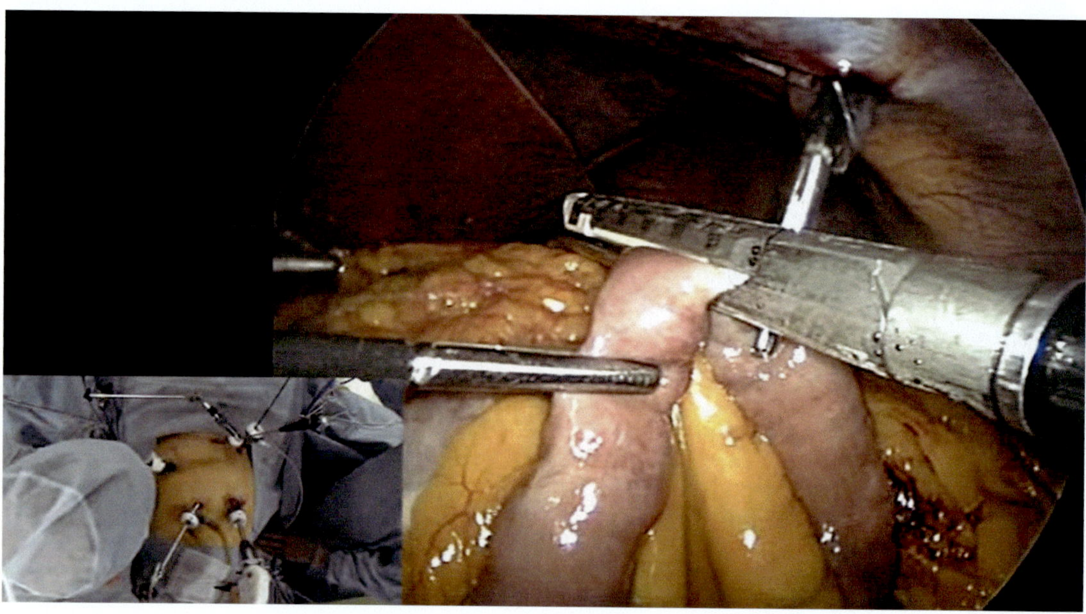

Fig. 10.6 The jejunum is transected 100 cm from the ligament of Traitz

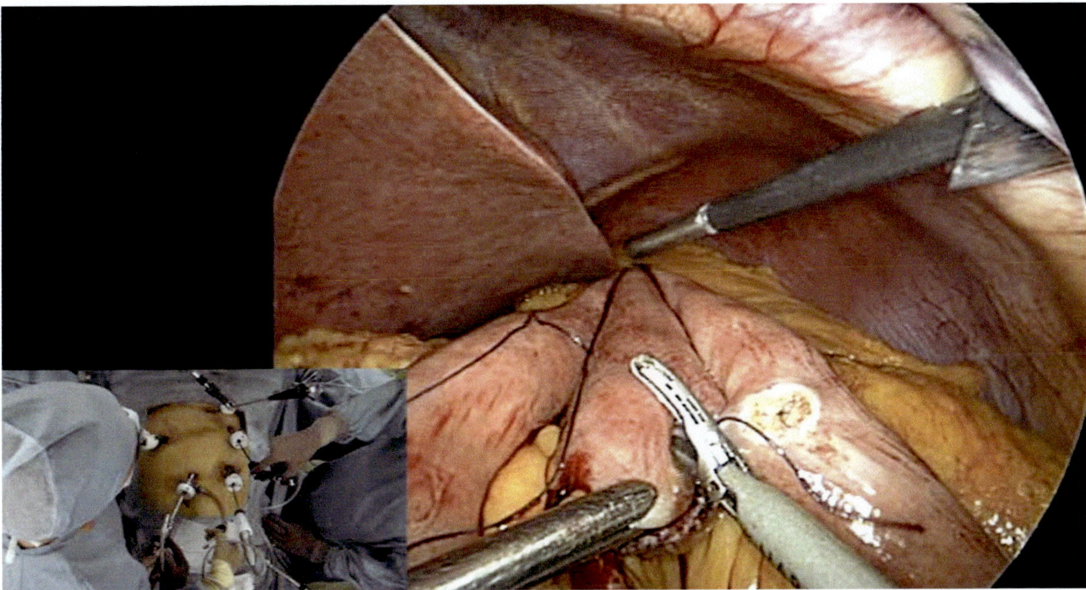

Fig. 10.7 After tow stay sutures are placed at the proximal and distal position of anastomosis, open the entry hole of the stapler

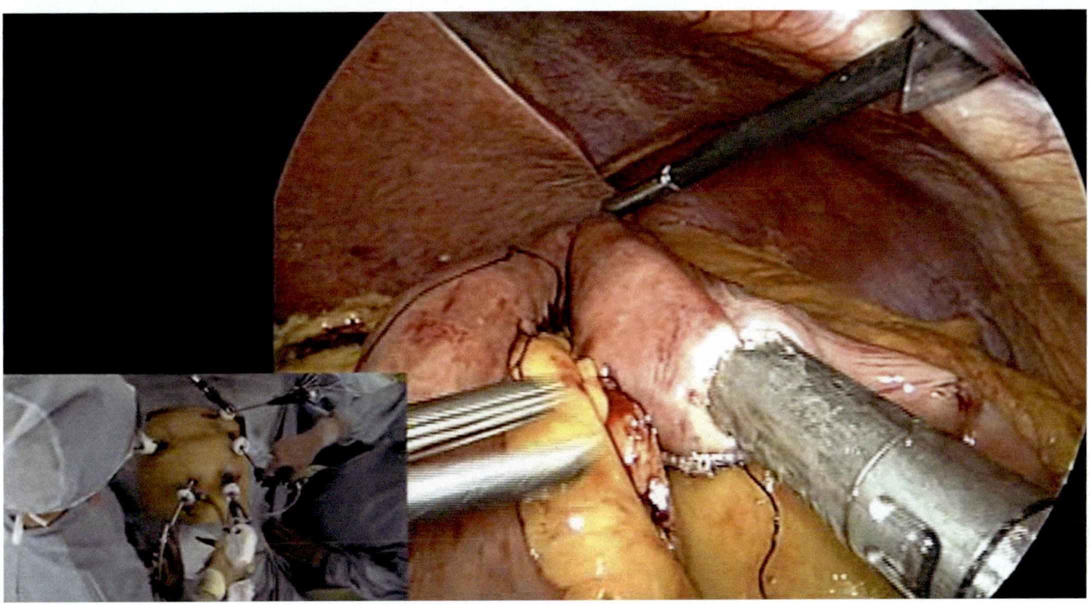

Fig. 10.8 A white 60 mm linear stapler is inserted through the hole to make the jejunojejunostomy

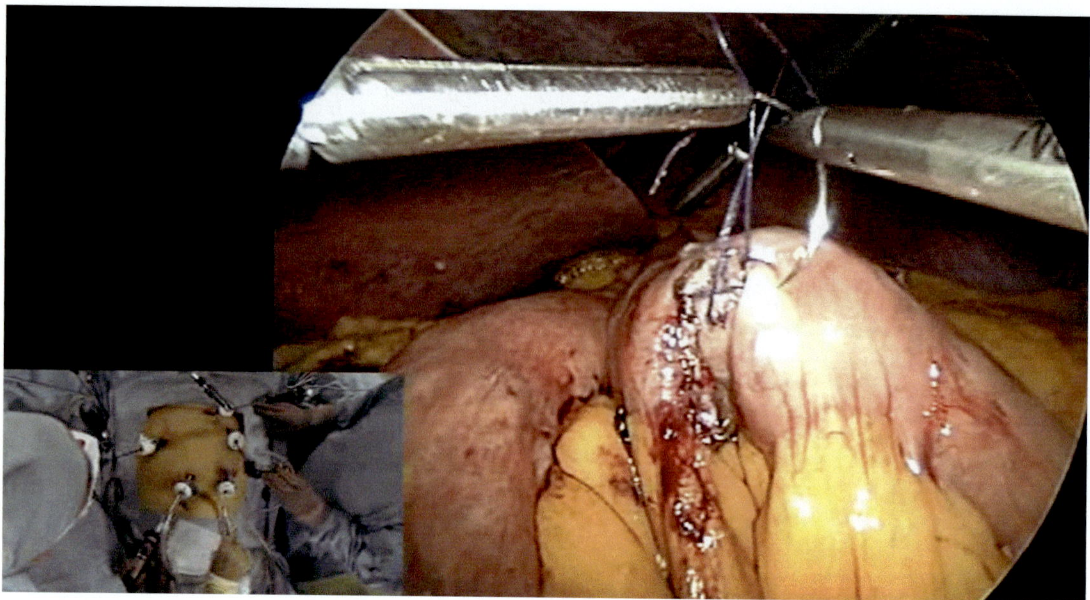

Fig. 10.9 The enterotomy is closed with a single layer of 3–0 absorbable suture

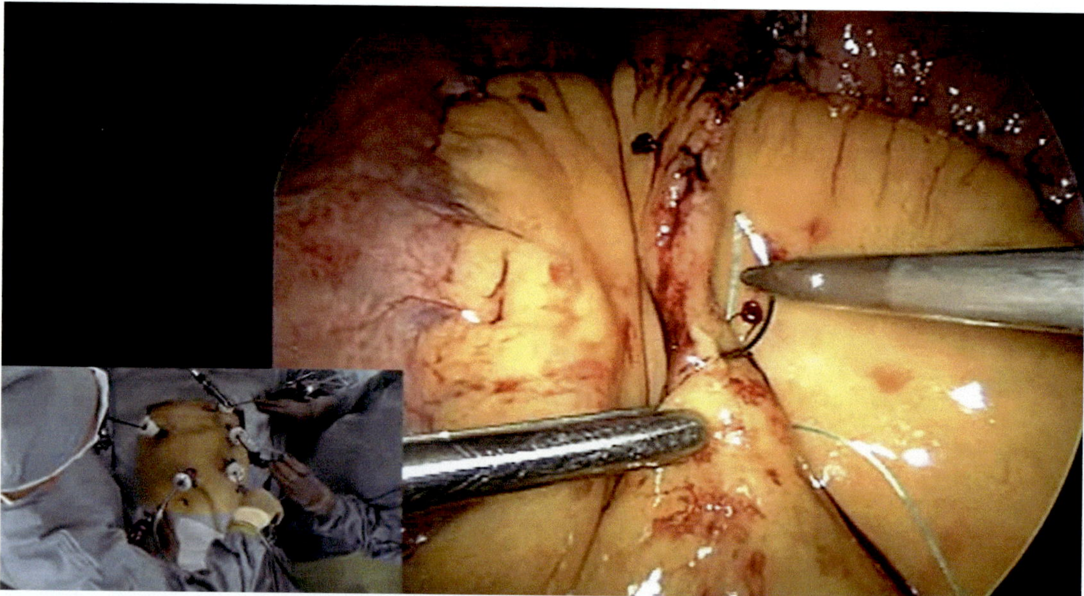

Fig. 10.10 Mesenteric defect closure

stapled anastomosis. If there is bleeding, it is helpful to use sutures. The enterotomy is closed with a single layer of 3-0 absorbable suture (Fig. 10.9). Use a continuous suture and tie it with the stay suture. The mesenteric defect must be closed with a continuous, nonabsorbable suture to limit the possibility of internal hernia (Fig. 10.10).

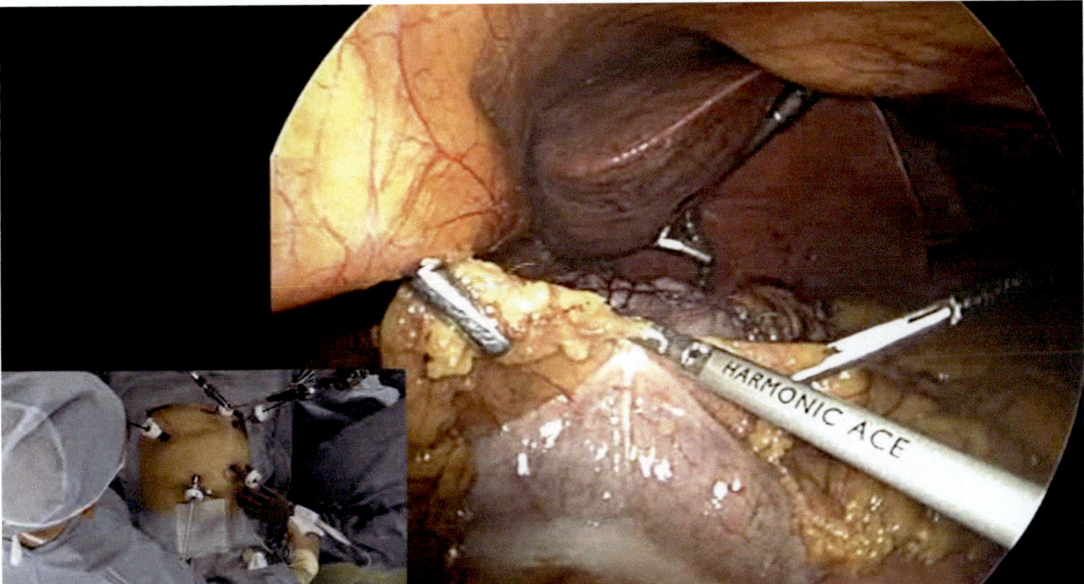

Fig. 10.11   Division of omentum

10.2.3 Duodenojejunostomy

As duodenojejunostomy is commonly performed using the antecolic method, the omentum should be divided with LCS to avoid the tension to the anastomosis (Fig. 10.11). Duodenojejunostomy is the most important part of this surgery. This anastomosis can be fashioned in several ways similar to the gastrojejunostomy in LRYGB, such as using a circular stapler, linear stapler, and hand suturing. We prefer to perform the hand suturing method with double layer anastomosis to reduce the risk of leakage. Other advantages of hand suturing anastomosis are described in the chapter of LRYGB.

First, a seromuscular suture is performed on the posterior wall between the oral side of the transected duodenum. The surgeon should be standing on the right side of the patient when the first stitch is made (Fig. 10.12). Then, the surgeon moves to the left side of the patient and the camera comes through the #4 port of Fig. 10.2, and the surgeon's hands manipulate his instruments through the ports #1 and #3 to keep the coaxial setting. Continuous suture of the posterior

seromuscular suture is performed with an absorbable suture (Fig. 10.13). Enterotomies are performed on the duodenum and the Roux limb adjacent to the suture line with LCS. A second posterior, full-thickness, running suture is performed continued anteriorly beyond the termination of the first posterior suture (Fig. 10.14). Two anterior suture lines are run from the distal anterior aspect of the enterotomy; the first is full thickness and tied with the full-thickness suture of the posterior wall (Fig. 10.15). The second anterior suture is seromuscular and tied with the seromuscular suture of the posterior wall (Fig. 10.16).

It is necessary to close the Petersen's space with a nonabsorbable suture to reduce the risk of internal hernia. After clamping the small intestine, perform a leak test with an endoscope (Fig. 10.17). The specimen of sleeve gastrectomy is retrieved through the 15 mm trocar site. The 15 mm trocar site should be closed, and the other trocar site may be closed if bleeding is detected on the site.

A drain is routinely used in our hospital, but its use depends on the surgeon's preference.

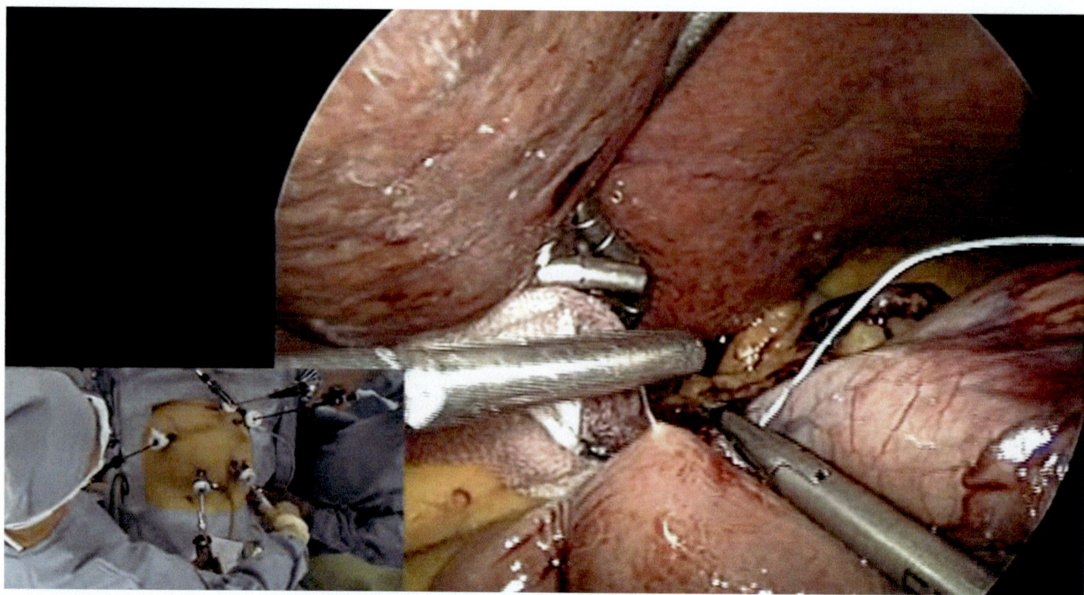

Fig 10.12 The first stitch of duodenojejunostomy

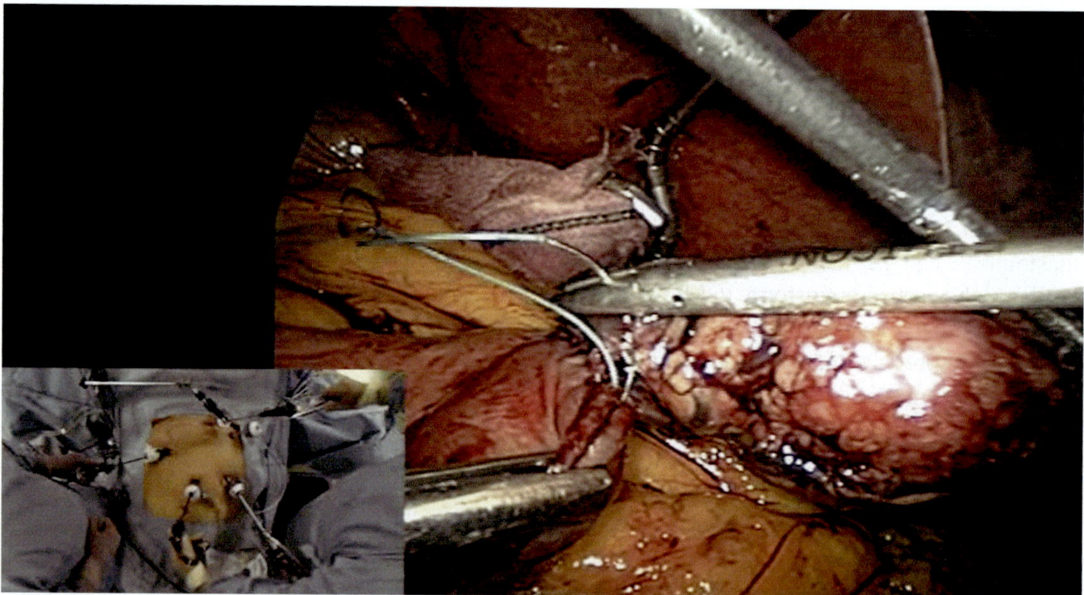

Fig. 10.13 Posterior seromuscular suturing

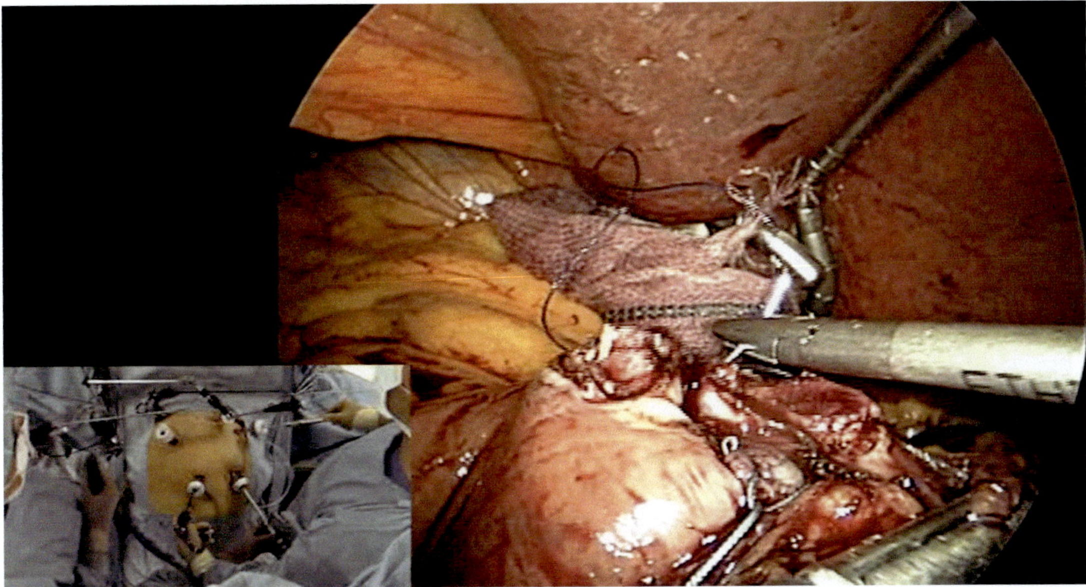

Fig. 10.14 Posterior full thickness suturing

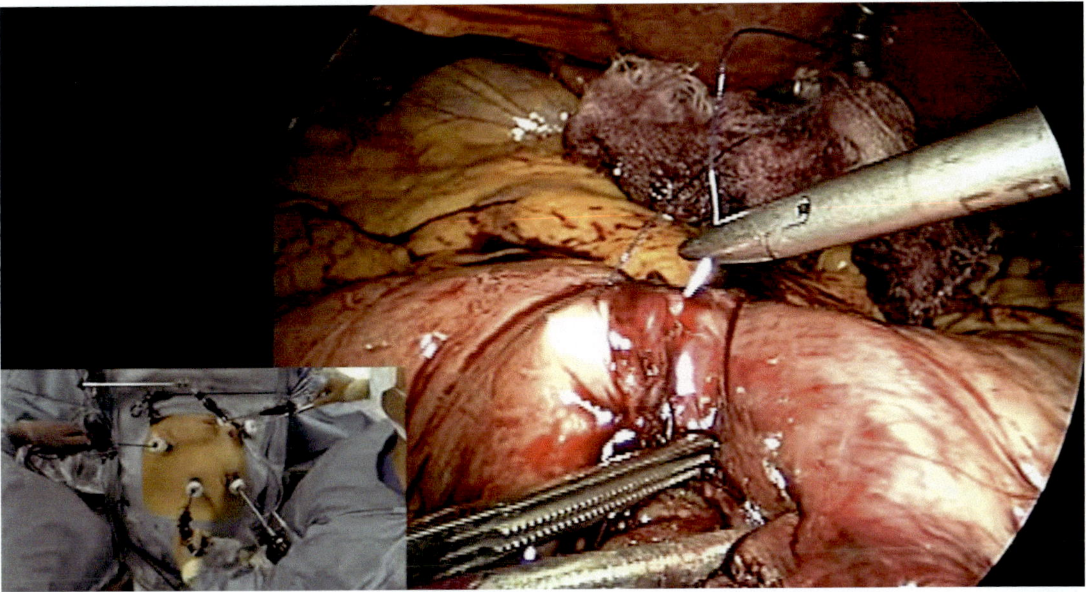

Fig. 10.15 Anterior full thickness suturing

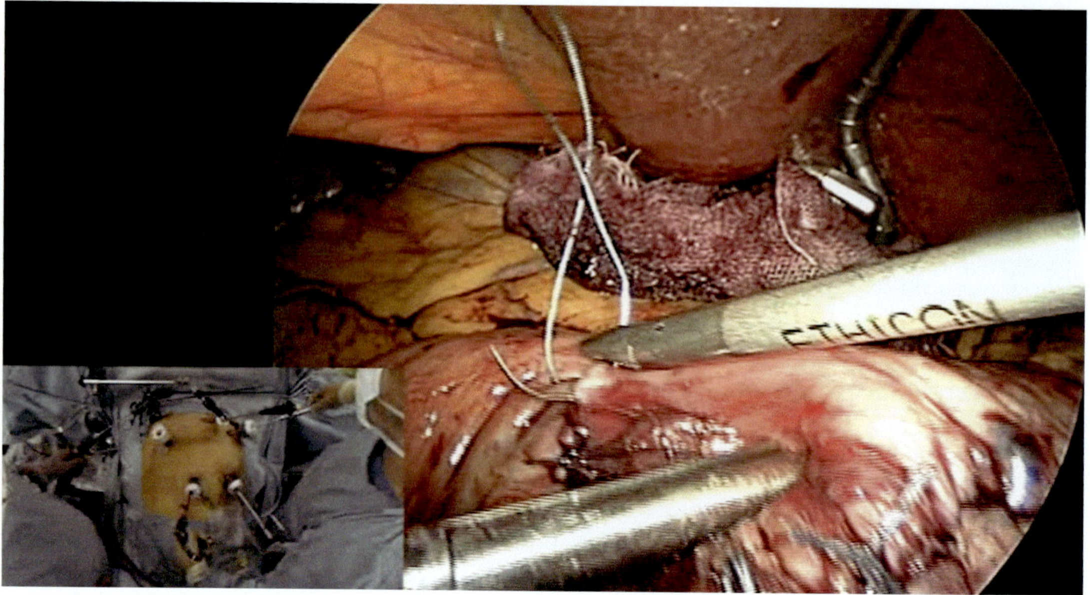

Fig. 10.16 Anterior seromuscular suturing

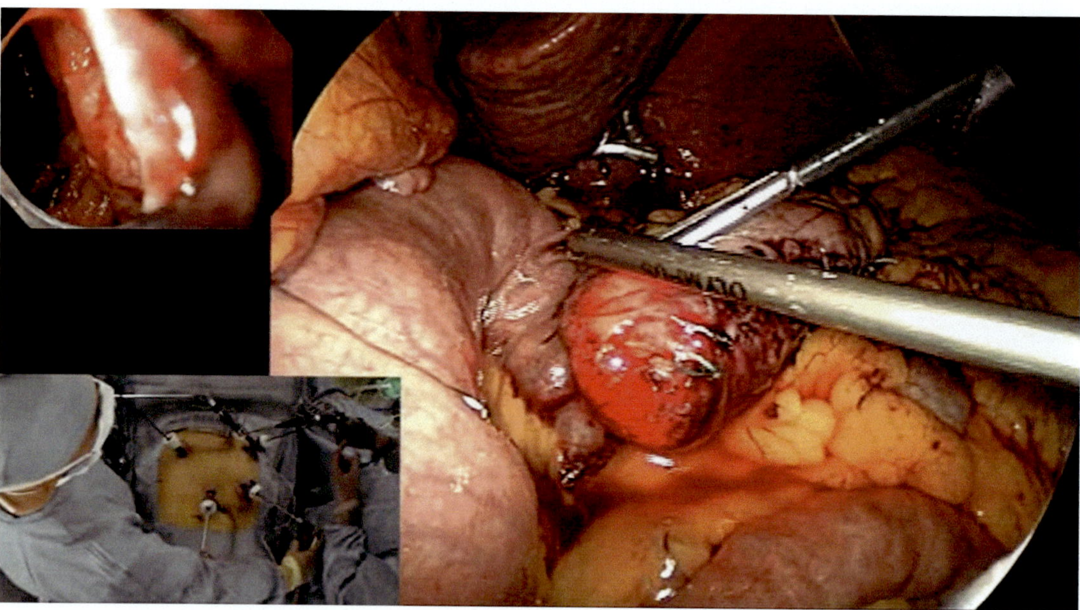

Fig. 10.17 Leak test with endoscope

10.3   Postoperative Considerations

Patients can receive a clear liquid diet on the first postoperative day after a water-soluble (gastrographine) upper gastrointestinal contrast test. The postoperative protocol for this procedure at our hospital is exactly same as LRYGB except the PPI (proton pomp inhibitor) doses. PPI is necessary after this operation for at least 1 month, similar to LSG. The drain is removed on the second postoperative day, and the patient can usually be discharged on the third postoperative day.

Further Videos

Electronic supplementary material is available in the online version of this chapter at (doi:10.1007/978-3-642-35591-2_10) and accessible for authorised users. Videos can also be accessed at http://www.springerimages.com/videos/978-3-642-35590-5

Reference

1. Kasama K, Tagaya N, Kanehira E. Laparoscopic sleeve gastrectomy with duodenojejunal bypass: technique and preliminary results. Obes Surg. 2009;19(10):1341–5.

Revisional Bariatric Surgery

11

Ji Yeon Park and Yong Jin Kim

11.1 Introduction

The World Health Organization (WHO) determined that obesity is a disease in need of long-term management in 1996. Obesity is closely related to various medical conditions including hypertension, diabetes, sleep apnea, dyslipidemia, gastroesophageal reflux disorder (GERD), arthropathy, and infertility, as well as malignancies such as breast and colorectal cancers. These conditions could be significantly improved or cured by losing weight. However, conventional conservative management with behavioral or medical options was unsatisfactory for achieving effective and sustained weight loss. Bariatric surgery is accepted as the only effective treatment for morbidly obese patients to reduce weight in the long term and improve obesity-related comorbidities at the same time [1, 2]. At present, there is no ideal bariatric procedure, and all bariatric surgical procedures have an associated failure rate requiring revisional surgery. As the bariatric surgery is becoming more and more prevalent, the number of patients asking for a solution for

weight regain or intolerable side effects after primary bariatric surgery is going to increase. Recently, revisional bariatric surgery comprises 10–25 % of total bariatric surgery [2, 3]. We here reviewed the preoperative evaluation before revisional surgery and proper choice among various reoperative options.

11.2 Indications for Revisional Bariatric Surgery

There are two major indications for revising a primary bariatric operation: insufficient weight loss or complications following primary bariatric surgery. There is no controversy over determining revisional surgery due to postoperative complications, but adequacy of weight loss must be judged based on the thorough evaluation. Before considering whether a particular individual is a candidate for a revision of the primary operation, it is important to determine whether there is an anatomic cause for the weight regain or the weight regain is primarily a result of behavioral discrepancies. Approximately 20 % of the patients who failed to obtain adequate weight loss following primary surgery might benefit from counseling with expert nutritionists or psychotherapists. It should also be considered and accepted that not everyone can be cured of their obesity; there is a group of nonresponders who are resistant to weight loss despite the surgeon's best efforts [4].

The rate of revisional surgery ranges from 0.76 to 40 % after gastric band [5], 10–20 % after gastric

J.Y. Park, MD • Y.J. Kim, MD, PhD (✉)
Department of Surgery, Soonchunhyang University Hospital, 59, Daesagwan-ro, Yongsan-gu, Seoul, 140-743, Republic of Korea
e-mail: yjgs1997@gmail.com

S.H. Choi, K. Kasama (eds.), *Bariatric and Metabolic Surgery*,
DOI 10.1007/978-3-642-35591-2_11, © Springer-Verlag Berlin Heidelberg 2014

bypass surgery [2, 6], and 5.5 % after sleeve gastrectomy [7]. Postoperative complications requiring secondary revisional surgery include the following: band slippage, erosion, stenosis, and port-related problems after adjustable gastric banding and bleeding from marginal ulcer, anastomotic stenosis, gastrogastric fistula after RYGB. Intolerable GERD is the most common cause requiring revisional surgery after sleeve gastrectomy [4, 6, 8, 9]. Selection for the surgical method of revision varies between cases. Adding malabsorptive procedure, such as Roux-en-Y gastric bypass or duodenal switch, is recommended after the purely restrictive surgery including adjustable gastric banding and sleeve gastrectomy. Distal RYGB or biliopancreatic diversion with duodenal switch can be followed by the initial RYGB decreasing the length of bypassed small bowel [1, 2, 4].

11.3 Preoperative Evaluation

11.3.1 Dietary Intake Diary and Nutrition Counseling

It is essential to evaluate and correct the inadequate dietary habit of the patient before revisional surgery, because most of these patients report the inability to eat appropriately in terms of food choices or adequate calories. Nutrition consultation is based on a food diary listing the patient's day-to-day dietary history. For some patients with weight regain or persistent nausea and vomiting, dietary modification alone can improve symptoms and control weight regain. Use of appetite suppressant for a certain period might be added to curb appetite and augment behavior modification in consequent. It is also necessary to investigate nutritional and metabolic status of the patients prior to revisional surgery.

11.3.2 Endoscopic Evaluation

Endoscopic evaluation is mandatory before revisional surgery. It can provide the important

diagnostic information of the previous surgery when the operation record is not available. Gastroesophageal reflux, marginal ulcer or stenosis, bleeding, and enteral fistula might be detected by endoscopy.

11.3.3 Contrast Upper GI Study (Fig. 11.1)

A contrast upper GI study could provide anatomic information of the gastrointestinal tract of the patient as well as the functional stenosis of fistula of the intestine. Furthermore, it also helps surgeon to understand postoperative status compared to preoperative status.

11.3.4 Other Studies

Manometry is useful to detect any influence from previous operation to esophageal peristalsis, and gastric emptying study might help to detect any functional abnormality.

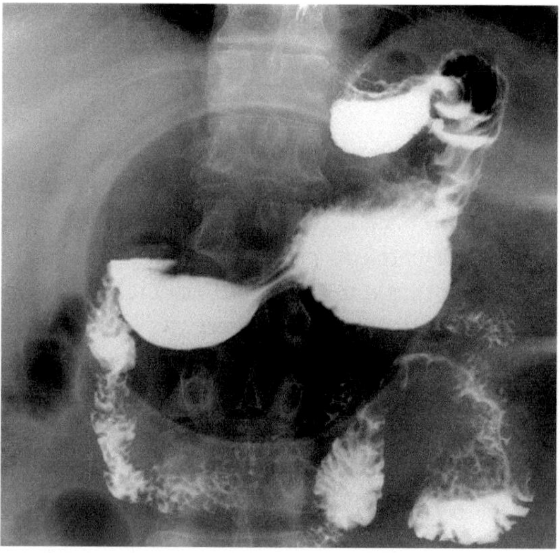

Fig. 11.1 Markedly large pouch noticed 30 months after sleeve gastrectomy, caused by dilatation of remnant stomach or left too big during the operation. This patient underwent revisional surgery to Roux-en-Y gastric bypass

11.3.5 Review of the Previous Operation Records

Reviewing the previous operation records is imperative, as anatomic anomaly or surgical techniques used in the previous surgery would substantially affect surgical strategy. When the primary surgical option was gastric bypass surgery, it is helpful to acknowledge the length of bypassed small bowel, the method of gastroje-junal anastomosis, whether the mesenteric defect had been repaired or not. In case of failed gastric banding, detailed information such as the type and the size of gastric band, any anatomic variations encountered on primary operation could be important.

11.3.6 Other Things to Check Before the Revisional Surgery

To avoid postoperative complications, any underlying diseases of the patient and the change after the primary operation should be noticed before revisional surgery. Preoperative work-up for deep vein thrombosis which can be precipitated by obesity or by other concurrent diseases is also necessary [10].

11.4 General Principles of the Revisional Bariatric Surgery

11.4.1 Adhesiolysis (Fig. 11.2)

Most of the revisional surgery can be performed via laparoscopic approach. Laparoscopic approach might be beneficial when the surgeon is used to laparoscopic procedures and fully understands the mechanism of adhesion even if the primary operation was performed via the open approach. Adhesion is generally encountered around the stomach (especially near to lesser curvature), liver, pancreas, left gastric artery, and inferior vena cava. If dense adhesion is present at the angle of His along the splenic hilum, up to the gastric fundus, careful adhesiolysis is necessary. Wider dissection than surgeon's initial judgment might be helpful to understand better about the anatomy of the previous operative field.

11.4.2 Utilizing Commercially Available Staplers

Staple loads with a staple height of 4.5 or 4.8 mm would be appropriate to use in gastric resection, because of thickened gastric wall secondary to edema and chronic inflammation from the primary

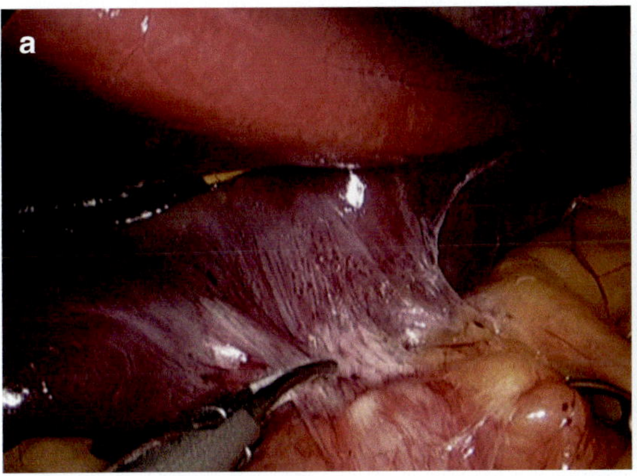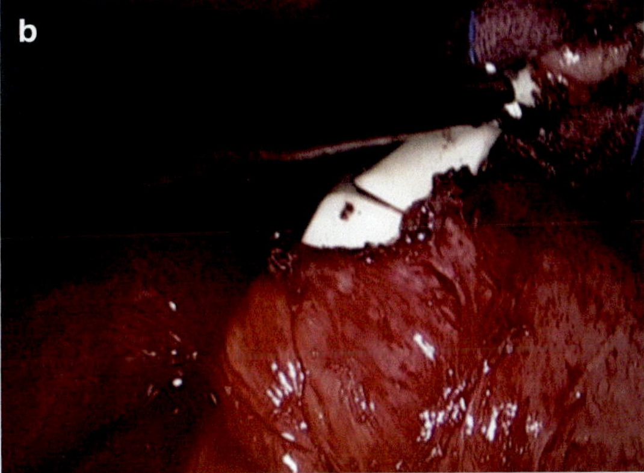

Fig. 11.2 Revision after adjustable gastric banding. (**a**) Severe adhesion around the lesser curvature between the stomach and liver. (**b**) Dissecting the adhesion around the band to isolate the band

surgery. The crossed section by stapling should always be carefully inspected for any evidence of bleeding and reinforced if needed.

11.4.3 Leak Test

The risk of leakage increases in the revisional surgery compared to the initial operation; therefore, the integrity of the anastomoses should be ensured before finishing the surgery. Methylene blue dye instillation or air insufflations via an endoscope or nasogastric tube are the most commonly used method to test for leakage. Endoscopic evaluation of the anastomosis site for any evidence of leak would be even safer, if it is available.

11.4.4 Gastrostomy

As the risk of gastrojejunal anastomotic leakage increases in revisional surgery, gastrostomy tube placement in the distal remnant pouch should be considered during Roux-en-Y gastric bypass as a revisional surgery [1–3]. It is also recommended to place gastrostomy tube into the remnant stomach when there is an evident nutritional deficiency or extensive adhesiolysis around the remnant stomach is required, which might cause postoperative distension of the remnant stomach.

11.4.5 Drains

It is the surgeons' choice whether to put drains into the abdominal cavity or not. However, when there is difficulty in making anastomosis or a repair is needed after leak test, intra-abdominal drains are highly recommended to form controlled fistula if a leak were to develop.

11.5 Revision After Adjustable Gastric Banding

11.5.1 Indications

There are several different reasons that cause failure of adjustable gastric banding. When pure technical problem such as gastric band slippage occurs, repositioning the original band or replacing it with the next-generation band would simply solve the problem. However, when the band had eroded into the stomach, the patient will be better managed by removing the band and converting to the other surgical options after a certain period of time [8, 11]. Abnormal esophageal motility, inadequate weight loss, development of GERD, and psychological intolerance are another reasons to consider conversion to another weight loss procedures [6, 11, 12]. There is no clear answer to the question that which procedure is preferred in certain circumstances after gastric banding failed. However, most of the previous studies suggested that conversion to the Roux-en-Y gastric bypass is superior to rebanding in patients with inadequate weight loss [12–14].

11.5.2 Surgical Procedures

11.5.2.1 Band Removal

Band removal is the easiest way to manage band failure. Band can be identified by following the band tube. Once the band is identified, adhesion around the band is carefully dissected to isolate the band. The band can be transected with laparoscopic scissors or ultrasonic shears. It has been reported that the adjustable gastric band eroded into the stomach cancer be safely removed endoscopically, although it is not a generalized practice yet [15].

11.5.2.2 Band Replacement

If the patient was showing good result with adequate weight loss after adjustable gastric banding, it is reasonable to perform band replacement for revision. However, conversion to other surgical procedures should be deliberately considered in patients with insufficient weight loss, recurrent erosion, and persistent intolerable nausea and vomiting after gastric banding. Careful selection among various options of revisional surgery is important to avoid additional postoperative complications as well as repetitive weight loss failure, and band replacement cannot bring about satisfactory weight loss in these patients [6, 11, 13]. Zundel et al. suggested that shifting the band to a different location after establishing a tract from the opposite direction is a safe method to avoid further adhesion and band slippage [16]. The fundus has to be unfolded completely to the normal anatomical location before band replacement to secure proper volume of the pouch and keep adequate positioning of the new band.

11.5.2.3 Adjustable Gastric Band Conversion to Sleeve Gastrectomy (Fig. 11.3)

Both of adjustable gastric band and sleeve gastrectomy are purely restrictive surgeries. Sleeve gastrectomy is a possible choice when patient has problems with band function in spite of adequate weight loss with adjustable gastric banding. The most common reasons include anatomic variations that preclude band replacement and the patient's low level of compliance with band adjustment. After removing the band, normal anatomy should be restored with sufficient dissection. Linear staplers with larger height than usual, such as 4.5 or 4.8 mm, should be considered as the gastric wall around fundus would be thickened due to the previous gastric banding operation. A few small retrospective studies reported on the short-term results of the sleeve gastrectomy which are converted from adjustable gastric banding. Foletto et al. reported 19.5 % of postoperative complications rate, 41.5 % of excess body weight loss in 2 years among 41 patients [17]. Iannelli et al. reported that among 36 patients who required revision to sleeve gastrectomy because of inadequate weight loss with adjustable gastric banding, postoperative complication rate was 12.2 % and excess weight loss was 42.7 % at mean follow-up period of 13.4 months. Six patients required further conversion to biliopancreatic diversion or Roux-en-Y gastric bypass eventually [18].

11.5.2.4 Adjustable Gastric Band Conversion to Roux-en-Y Gastric Bypass (Fig. 11.4)

Indications for conversion from adjustable gastric banding to Roux-en-Y gastric bypass include the following: patient's psychological intolerance with band, inadequate weight loss after adjustable gastric banding, when intolerable gastroesophageal reflux disease or esophageal dysmotility occurred. Normal gastric anatomy should be restored before making gastric pouch to optimize the volume of the pouch. Careful dissection should be carried out along the lesser curvature and around cardia, and also at the angle of His where adhesion cannot be avoided. Van Wageningen et al. reported the results of the 47 patients who underwent conversion from AGB to RYGB [19]. The early complication rate was 17 %, and one patient developed incisional hernia in the late period. Mean follow-up period was 5 years and 6 months after initial surgery, while 12 months after revisional surgery. Mean BMI was 49.2 ± 9.3 kg/m^2 before undergoing AGB,

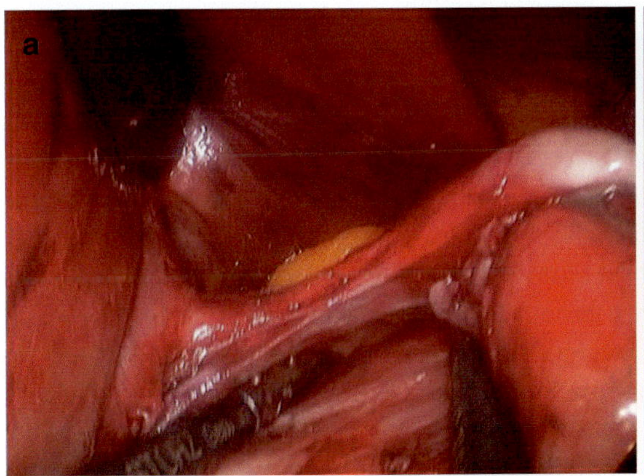
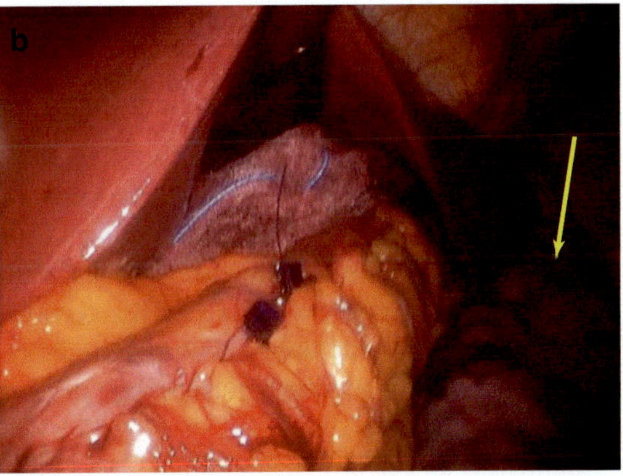

Fig. 11.3 Revisional surgery to sleeve gastrectomy following adjustable gastric banding. (**a**) Careful dissection of adhesion along the lesser curvature. (**b**) The stomach was fully transected with linear staplers, and staple line was oversewn with running sutures. Resected stomach is marked with *arrow*

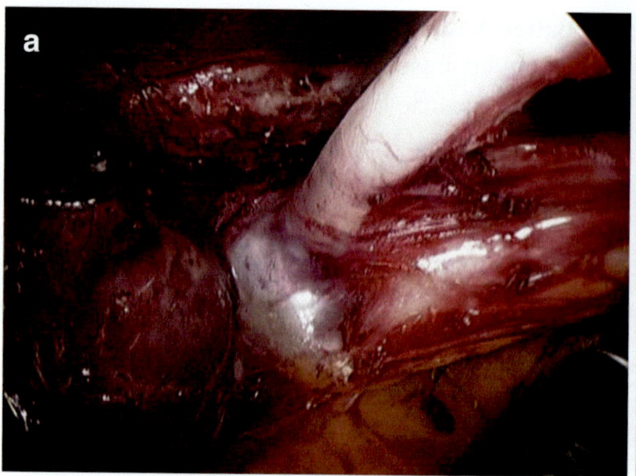
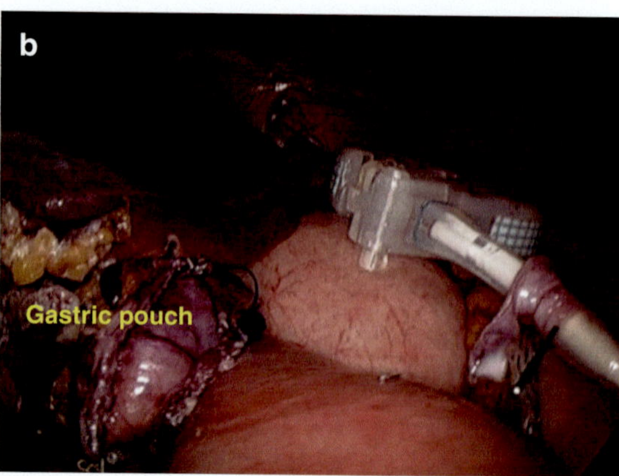

Fig. 11.4 Adjustable gastric banding converted to Roux-en-Y gastric bypass. (**a**) Severe adhesion around the band. (**b**) Final situation after completion of the antecolic Roux-en-Y gastric bypass with creation of a mini-gastric pouch. Removed band is seen on the right

45.8 ± 8.9 kg/m² after gastric banding, and 37.7 ± 8.7 kg/m² after conversion to RYGB.

Mognol et al. analyzed 70 patients who underwent conversion of AGB to RYGB [14]. The early complication rate was 14.3 %, which included intraluminal bleeding and wound infection. Late major complication developed in 8.6 % of the patients, which were 3 gastrojejunal anastomotic stenosis and 3 marginal ulcers. Mean excess weight loss was 70 % and mean BMI decreased from 44.9 ± 10.8 to 32.2 ± 6.3 kg/m² during the 18 months after revisional surgery.

11.6 Revisional Surgery After Sleeve Gastrectomy (Fig. 11.5)

The most common causes for revisional surgery after sleeve gastrectomy are insufficient weight loss and GERD. Additional sleeve gastrectomy [18] or conversion to RYGB [19] can be considered for inadequate weight loss. The incidence of GERD following sleeve gastrectomy is reported at 5–36 % [7], and conversion to RYGB is recommended when the symptom or abnormal findings at esophagogastric junction persist despite proper medical treatment [9].

Iannelli et al. performed additional sleeve gastrectomy between October 2005 and April 2010 in 13 patients who showed insufficient weight

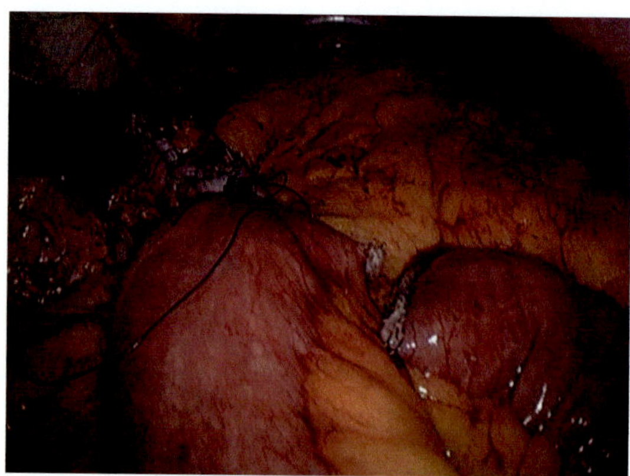

Fig. 11.5 Final configuration after revision of sleeve gastrectomy converted to Roux-en-Y gastric bypass. After creating gastric pouch, jejunum was brought upward to the stomach to create gastrojejunostomy and then divided to prevent bile reflux

loss or regained weight after initial sleeve gastrectomy [20]. The initial mean BMI and excess weight loss were 44.6(37–52.9) kg/m² and 61.8 kg. Mean BMI after secondary sleeve gastrectomy was 32.3 kg/m² at 1 month, 32 kg/m² at 6 months, 27.5 kg/m² at 12 months, and excess weight loss was 50.3, 47.9, and 71.4 % at each time points. Van Rutte et al. reported that 23 patients were converted to RYGB among 676 patients who underwent sleeve gastrectomy between 2006 and 2011 [7]. Mean BMI was 34.4 (25.6–46.2) kg/m², and excess weight loss was

52.5 % (8.9–85.9) at 12 months after revisional surgery in these patients.

Gautier et al. reported that 18 patients required conversion of sleeve gastrectomy to RYGB for several reasons: inadequate weight loss in 9 patients, intolerable GERD in 3 patients, and persistent diabetes in 3 patients [21]. Excess weight loss increased from 47.1 % before revisional surgery to 6 [22] 4.6 % at 15 months after revisional RYGB. The reflux symptom disappeared in all patients with GERD, and patients with diabetes discontinued to take hypoglycemic medications. There was one complication of small bowel injury.

11.7 Revisional Surgery Following RYGB

11.7.1 Indications

Insufficient weight loss or weight regain is reported to occur in 15–25 % of the patients following RYGB [23–25]. When behavioral pattern rather than anatomic problem caused the failure, revisional surgery is not indicated. Therefore, thorough nutritional and psychological counseling is imperative before deciding to undertake revisional surgery. The common causes for revisional surgery following RYGB include marginal ulcers, gastric fistula, gastrojejunostomy site stenosis, or obstruction.

11.7.2 Options for Revisional Surgery and Their Outcomes

11.7.2.1 Addition of Restrictive Procedure

It is controversial to perform additional restrictive procedure for patients with inadequate weight loss or weight regain after initial RYGB. Theoretically, if an enlarged gastric pouch or gastrojejunal stoma is responsible for the failure, adding restriction could be a reasonable solution. Both of the gastric pouch and gastrojejunostomy can be revised to reduce the size, or AGB can be additionally applied at gastric pouch near the anastomosis [26]. Additional AGB has

advantages of avoiding the risks following revision of the anastomosis while increasing restriction. Gastrogastric fixation of the AGB using the remnant stomach is the common technique to prevent postoperative band slippage.

Bessler et al. reported that 22 patients who underwent additional AGB after RYGB failure showed 47 % of mean excess weight loss at 5 years [26]. The other study by Gobble et al. assessing AGB after RYGB failure consisted of 11 patients with mean BMI of 43.4 kg/m^2. The mean BMI after revision was 37.1 kg/m^2, and they showed additional 20.8 % of mean excess weight loss over the mean follow-up period of 13 months, which led to total 59 % of EWL eventually [27].

Another procedure of restriction, sleeve gastrectomy, can be added to the failed RYGB. However, Parikh et al. reported that 14 patients revised with sleeve gastrectomy due to inadequate weight loss after RYGB did not show significant weight loss during the 1 year follow-up period [22].

Recently developed technique includes endoscopic sclerotherapy, which is performed by injecting sodium morrhuate into the rim of GJ anastomosis, and gastrojejunal sleeve reduction, although they are not introduced in Korea yet [22, 28].

11.7.3 Addition of Malabsorptive Procedures

11.7.3.1 Conversion to Distal RYGB

Malabsorption can be added by increasing the length of Roux limb or biliopancreatic limb after RYGB. Conversion to a distal RYGB with long limb can be considered when the patient has the Roux limb less than 150 cm and normal anatomy of gastrojejunostomy (i.e., gastric pouch less than 30 ml and a stoma less than 15 mm). This procedure is known to be relatively simple from the technical point of view as difficult dissection at upper abdomen is unnecessary. Common channel is usually measured from ileocecal valve toward proximally, although the approach can vary. The length of common channel typically ranges from

75 to 150 cm, which is critical. A length less than 75 cm is inappropriate and has a high risk of protein malnutrition [29].

Sugerman et al. published the results of 27 patients who underwent distal RYGB converted from proximal RYGB. The length of Roux limb was 40–145 cm with 50 cm-length common channel in the initial 5 patients, and the other 22 patients had 150 cm-long common channel [30]. The initial 5 patients suffered from severe protein malnutrition and nutritional deficiency and required reoperation eventually. Two of them died of hepatic failure. Of the 22 patients with 150 cm common channel, 3 patients required revision due to malnutrition. All the patients showed nutritional deficiency in at least 1 category by blood tests, and 4 of them (18 %) required total parenteral nutrition. The EWL at 5 years was 69 %, and most of the comorbidities were resolved 1 year after the revisional surgery.

Fobi et al. performed conversion to distal RYGB by moving the Roux limb distally halfway down the common channel, reducing the length of alimentary limb by 50 % in 65 patients [31]. These patients showed the mean body weight and BMI loss of 20 kg additionally after the revisional surgery 7 kg/m^2. Intractable diarrhea developed in 3 %, and nutritional support was necessary via gastrostomy in eight patients and with total parenteral nutrition in six patients. Six of them required reoperation.

11.7.3.2 Conversion of RYGB to Biliopancreatic Diversion with Duodenal Switch

Duodenal switch can be conducted after RYGB failure, and the reported EWL ranges from 15 to 20 % [2, 3, 32, 33]. However, biliopancreatic diversion and duodenal switch is a complicated procedure which requires 3 or 4 anastomoses: gastrogastrostomy, duodenoileostomy, and jejunojejunostomy. This technically challenging procedure can be performed in 1 or 2 stages by open or laparoscopic surgery.

The indication for conversion of RYGB to BPD-DS is still controversial, but reactive hypoglycemia can be the one reason. When a patient is not compliant with low-carbohydrate diet, recreating the pylorus can relieve the reactive hypoglycemic symptoms by delaying carbohydrate passage into small bowel [34].

The studies on duodenal switch followed by RYGB failure are extremely scarce. Greenbaum et al. reported the results from 41 patients who were converted to duodenal switch after RYGB [35]. The mean EWL after revisional surgery was 54 % in 25 patients at 6 months, 59 % in 15 patients at 1 year, and 77 % in 5 patients at 2 years. The incidence of major complication was 32 %, and there was no mortality.

Keshishian et al. first reported on the conversion of RYGB to BPD-DS [36]. This study included 47 patients who had revisional surgery, and three-fourths of the patients underwent BPD-DS as a revisional procedure due to inadequate weight loss or weight regain (46 %) or intolerable dumping syndrome (28 %). The incidence of leakage was 8.5 %, and mean BMI decreased from 48.9 to 29.2 kg/m^2, mean EWL was 67 %, and mean body weight loss was 48 kg over 30 months of follow-up period. The primary problems that resulted in revisions were resolved in all patients [36].

Conclusion

Bariatric surgery has been increasingly performed over the last half century as its efficacy and safety are demonstrated. Thus, the demand on revisional surgery also increases due to surgical complications or inadequate weight loss after the initial surgery. However, revisional surgery does not always bring about good results in the long term. Thorough anatomic evaluation is essential before revisional surgery. Patient needs to make an effort to correct the behavioral problems during certain period of time before revisional surgery through deliberate counseling.

Revisional bariatric surgery is known to have a higher complication rate compared to the primary surgery. However, it is possible to achieve favorable outcomes regarding patient's quality of life and postoperative complications with careful selection of the indicated patients according to the surgeon's experience, thorough preoperative evaluation, and proper selection for the revisional method.

Further Videos

Electronic supplementary material is available in the online version of this chapter at (doi:10.1007/978-3-642-35591-2_11) and accessible for authorised users. Videos can also be accessed at http://www.springerimages.com/videos/978-3-642-35590-5

References

1. Kellogg TA. Revisional bariatric surgery. Surg Clin North Am. 2011;91(6):1353–71, x.
2. Radtka 3rd JF, Puleo FJ, Wang L, et al. Revisional bariatric surgery: who, what, where, and when? Surg Obes Relat Dis. 2010;6(6):635–42.
3. Hamoui N, Chock B, Anthone GJ, et al. Revision of the duodenal switch: indications, technique, and outcomes. J Am Coll Surg. 2007;204(4):603–8.
4. Jones Jr KB. Revisional bariatric surgery – potentially safe and effective. Surg Obes Relat Dis. 2005;1(6):599 603.
5. Singhal R, Bryant C, Kitchen M, et al. Band slippage and erosion after laparoscopic gastric banding: a meta-analysis. Surg Endosc. 2010;24(12):2980–6.
6. DeMaria EJ, Sugerman HJ, Meador JG, et al. High failure rate after laparoscopic adjustable silicone gastric banding for treatment of morbid obesity. Ann Surg. 2001;233(6):809–18.
7. van Rutte PW, Smulders JF, de Zoete JP, et al. Indications and short-term outcomes of revisional surgery after failed or complicated sleeve gastrectomy. Obes Surg. 2012;22(12):1903–8.
8. Gagner M, Gumbs AA. Gastric banding: conversion to sleeve, bypass, or DS. Surg Endosc. 2007;21(11). 1931–5.
9. Lacy A, Ibarzabal A, Pando E, et al. Revisional surgery after sleeve gastrectomy. Surg Laparosc Endosc Percutan Tech. 2010;20(5):351–6.
10. Inabnet 3rd WB, Belle SH, Bessler M, et al. Comparison of 30-day outcomes after non-LapBand primary and revisional bariatric surgical procedures from the Longitudinal Assessment of Bariatric Surgery study. Surg Obes Relat Dis. 2010;6(1):22–30.
11. Weber M, Muller MK, Michel JM, et al. Laparoscopic Roux-en-Y gastric bypass, but not rebanding, should be proposed as rescue procedure for patients with failed laparoscopic gastric banding. Ann Surg. 2003;238(6):827–33; discussion 833–4.
12. Suter M. Laparoscopic band repositioning for pouch dilatation/slippage after gastric banding: disappointing results. Obes Surg. 2001;11(4):507–12.
13. Westling A, Ohrvall M, Gustavsson S. Roux-en-Y gastric bypass after previous unsuccessful gastric restrictive surgery. J Gastrointest Surg. 2002;6(2):206–11.
14. Mognol P, Chosidow D, Marmuse JP. Laparoscopic conversion of laparoscopic gastric banding to Roux-en-Y gastric bypass: a review of 70 patients. Obes Surg. 2004;14(10):1349–53.
15. Neto MP, Ramos AC, Campos JM, et al. Endoscopic removal of eroded adjustable gastric band: lessons learned after 5 years and 78 cases. Surg Obes Relat Dis. 2010;6(4):423–7.
16. Zundel N, Hernandez JD. Revisional surgery after restrictive procedures for morbid obesity. Surg Laparosc Endosc Percutan Tech. 2010;20(5):338–43.
17. Foletto M, Prevedello L, Bernante P, et al. Sleeve gastrectomy as revisional procedure for failed gastric banding or gastroplasty. Surg Obes Relat Dis. 2010;6(2):146–51.
18. Iannelli A, Schneck AS, Ragot E, et al. Laparoscopic sleeve gastrectomy as revisional procedure for failed gastric banding and vertical banded gastroplasty. Obes Surg. 2009;19(9):1216–20.
19. van Wageningen B, Berends FJ, Van Ramshorst B, et al. Revision of failed laparoscopic adjustable gastric banding to Roux-en-Y gastric bypass. Obes Surg. 2006;16(2):137–41.
20. Iannelli A, Schneck AS, Noel P, et al. Re-sleeve gastrectomy for failed laparoscopic sleeve gastrectomy: a feasibility study. Obes Surg. 2011;21(7):832–5.
21. Gautier T, Sarcher T, Contival N, et al. Indications and mid-term results of conversion from sleeve gastrectomy to Roux-en-Y gastric bypass. Obes Surg. 2013;23(2):212–5.
22. Parikh M, Heacock L, Gagner M. Laparoscopic "gastrojejunal sleeve reduction" as a revision procedure for weight loss failure after Roux-en-Y gastric bypass. Obes Surg. 2011;21(5):650–4.
23. Sugerman HJ, Starkey JV, Birkenhauer R. A randomized prospective trial of gastric bypass versus vertical banded gastroplasty for morbid obesity and their

effects on sweets versus non-sweets eaters. Ann Surg. 1987;205(6):613–24.

24. Hall JC, Watts JM, O'Brien PE, et al. Gastric surgery for morbid obesity. The Adelaide Study. Ann Surg. 1990;211(4):419–27.

25. Lechner GW, Callender AK. Subtotal gastric exclusion and gastric partitioning: a randomized prospective comparison of one hundred patients. Surgery. 1981;90(4):637–44.

26. Bessler M, Daud A, DiGiorgi MF, et al. Adjustable gastric banding as revisional bariatric procedure after failed gastric bypass – intermediate results. Surg Obes Relat Dis. 2010;6(1):31–5.

27. Gobble RM, Parikh MS, Greives MR, et al. Gastric banding as a salvage procedure for patients with weight loss failure after Roux-en-Y gastric bypass. Surg Endosc. 2008;22(4):1019–22.

28. Abu Dayyeh BK, Jirapinyo P, Weitzner Z, et al. Endoscopic sclerotherapy for the treatment of weight regain after Roux-en-Y gastric bypass: outcomes, complications, and predictors of response in 575 procedures. Gastrointest Endosc. 2012;76(2):275–82.

29. Brolin RE, LaMarca LB, Kenler HA, et al. Malabsorptive gastric bypass in patients with superobesity. J Gastrointest Surg. 2002;6(2):195–203; discussion 204–5.

30. Sugerman HJ, Kellum JM, DeMaria EJ. Conversion of proximal to distal gastric bypass for failed gastric bypass for superobesity. J Gastrointest Surg. 1997; 1(6):517–24; discussion 524–6.

31. Fobi MA, Lee H, Igwe Jr D, et al. Revision of failed gastric bypass to distal Roux-en-Y gastric bypass: a review of 65 cases. Obes Surg. 2001;11(2): 190–5.

32. Zingg U, McQuinn A, DiValentino D, et al. Revisional vs. primary Roux-en-Y gastric bypass – a case-matched analysis: less weight loss in revisions. Obes Surg. 2010;20(12):1627–32.

33. Gagner M. Laparoscopic revisional surgery after malabsorptive procedures in bariatric surgery, more specifically after duodenal switch. Surg Laparosc Endosc Percutan Tech. 2010;20(5):344–7.

34. Kellogg TA, Bantle JP, Leslie DB, et al. Postgastric bypass hyperinsulinemic hypoglycemia syndrome: characterization and response to a modified diet. Surg Obes Relat Dis. 2008;4(4): 492–9.

35. Greenbaum DF, Wasser SH, Riley T, et al. Duodenal switch with omentopexy and feeding jejunostomy – a safe and effective revisional operation for failed previous weight loss surgery. Surg Obes Relat Dis. 2011; 7(2):213–8.

36. Keshishian A, Zahriya K, Hartoonian T, et al. Duodenal switch is a safe operation for patients who have failed other bariatric operations. Obes Surg. 2004;14(9):1187–92.

Susumu Inamine

12.1 Introduction

Although the vast majority of bariatric procedures achieve successful outcomes and provide many benefits to the patients, there is still a significant risk of postoperative complications. Weight loss surgery is a relatively simple procedure that modifies the route of digestive tract. However, there are bariatric surgery specific complications different from that of other gastrointestinal procedures such as gastric cancer surgeries.

This chapter will review the major complications of weight loss surgery, focusing on the four standard procedures performed worldwide: laparoscopic Roux-en-Y gastric bypass (LRYGB), laparoscopic sleeve gastrectomy (LSG), laparoscopic adjustable gastric band (LAGB), and laparoscopic biliopancreatic diversion or duodenal switch (LBPD/DS).

Today, as most weight loss surgery is performed using laparoscopy, I will describe the complications connected to laparoscopic weight loss surgery.

General Aspects of Complications Connected to Bariatric Surgery The complications that develop following weight loss surgery vary based on the type of the procedures used. Surgery with internal anastomosis such as RYGB and BPD-DS has risks similar to that of other major abdominal operations

that include a gastrointestinal anastomosis. Operations such as LAGB may have lower complication rates, because the gastrointestinal tract is not opened. The complication rate of LSG has been reported to be between that of RYGB and LAGB.

12.2 Mortality

The overall 30-day mortality for bariatric surgical procedures varies in medical literature and by the type of procedure. The average statistics are 0.1 % for LAGB, 0.3 % for LSG, 0.5 % for gastric bypass, and 1.1 % for BPD/DS. These values compare favorably with the hospital mortality rates of other major surgical procedures including hip replacement (0.3 %), abdominal aneurysm repair (3.9 %), and pancreatic resection (8.3 %). The most common cause of early mortality is pulmonary emboli and complications related to leaks.

Factors associated with increased mortality risks are older age (>65 years), male gender, super obesity (BMI > 50), low-volume surgeons and hospitals (<100 procedures/year), and the use of open procedures (LRYGB:RYGB = 0.17 %:0.79 %).

12.3 Morbidity

The type of procedure affects the morbidity rate. The rate of morbidity following LAGB appears to be less than as seen with LRYGB in terms of major complications (1 % versus 3.3 %) within 30 days of the procedure. The patients who

S. Inamine, MD
Department of Endoscopic Surgery, Nakagami
General Hospital, Okinawa, Japan
e-mail: soohs@mac.com

S.H. Choi, K. Kasama (eds.), *Bariatric and Metabolic Surgery*,
DOI 10.1007/978-3-642-35591-2_12, © Springer-Verlag Berlin Heidelberg 2014

underwent open surgery had higher rates of complications compared to the patient who underwent laparoscopic surgery (7.4 % versus 3.4 %).

12.4 Common Intraoperative Complications in Bariatric Procedures

12.4.1 Trocar Injury

Trocar placement, especially first abdominal access in severely obese patients, can be difficult and dangerous because of the fairly thick abdominal wall. Many structures (abdominal wall vessels, the large or small intestine, mesentery vessels, aorta, vena cava, etc.) are at risk of injury during the introduction of the trocar, and some injuries such as damage of retroperitoneal vessels and mesenteric vessels can be life-threatening. Although there are three main techniques for first trocar insertion – Veress needle technique, Hasson's blunt trocar, and direct trocar insertion with optical view – there is no evidence as to the safest method. Some researchers advocate that trocar injury can be minimized by using the left upper quadrant as the first access site for the introduction of the trocars.

12.4.2 Splenic Injury

The spleen can also be injured during bariatric procedures, especially during LSG. It is sometimes difficult to control the bleeding from the spleen so particular attention must be paid to not injure the spleen while performing a dissection around the spleen.

12.5 Early Postoperative Complications

Possible early complications include bleeding, leaks, deep vein thrombosis, pulmonary embolism, and cardiovascular and pulmonary complications. Surgical experience may influence the complication rate. The learning curve for LRYGB may be as high as 100 cases.

12.5.1 Bleeding

Significant bleeding after gastric bypass has been reported in 0.6–4.0 % of patients.

Early bleeding typically occurs in intra- or extraluminal regions (intraluminal > extraluminal) from the site of anastomosis and/or staple lines. Patients frequently have tachycardia, decreased hematocrit levels, and melena. Such bleeding typically resolves without surgical intervention but may require the transfusion of blood products. Surgery should be reserved for cases with hemodynamic instability.

12.5.2 Wound Infection

The rates of wound infection are significantly higher with open (10–15 %) than laparoscopic (3–4 %) procedures. The incidence of wound infection can be reduced by the perioperative administration of antibiotic agents.

12.5.3 Pulmonary Embolism and Deep Venous Thrombosis

Pulmonary embolism (PE) remains the most common cause of patient mortality after bariatric surgery and can account for more than 50 % of deaths. A diagnosis of PE in morbidly obese patients can be problematic, because the use of standard diagnostic modalities may not be physically feasible in extremely obese patients. Immediate anticoagulation is prescribed for patients for whom there is high level of clinical suspicion. For patients in whom anticoagulation is contraindicated, a mechanical filter can be placed in the inferior vena cava to lower the risk of continued clot embolization. The optimal strategies for preventing DVT/PE in the gastric bypass setting have not been established. Most bariatric surgeons use both pneumatic compression devices in conjunction with subcutaneous unfractionated or low-molecular-weight heparin.

12.5.4 Cardiovascular Complications

Cardiovascular complications, including myocardial infarction and cardiac failure, are also common causes of mortality in the perioperative period. Mortality from cardiovascular events ranged from 12.5 to 17.6 %.

12.5.5 Pulmonary Complications

Respiratory failure accounts for 11.3 % of the perioperative mortality after weight loss surgery. Atelectasis is common after all types of surgery that require general anesthesia and is even more prevalent in the morbidly obese. Early ambulation and incentive spirometry after surgery are important to decrease the incidence of pulmonary complications. Preoperative identification of the presence of obstructive sleep apnea syndrome (OSAS) and the initiation of continuous positive airway pressure (CPAP) therapy also reduce the risk of pulmonary complications during the postoperative period.

12.5.6 Ventral Incisional Hernia

Ventral incisional hernias occur with a frequency of 0–1.8 % in both laparoscopic and open series, underscoring a clear advantage of the laparoscopic approach in this regard.

12.6 Late Complications

The late complications of bariatric surgery include cholelithiasis, nutritional deficiencies, and neurologic and psychiatric complications.

12.7 Complications of Specific Bariatric Procedures

12.7.1 Roux-en-Y Gastric Bypass

RYGB involves the creation of a small gastric pouch and an anastomosis to a Roux limb of the jejunum that bypasses 75–150 cm of the small bowel, thereby restricting food intake and limiting absorption. This procedure is the most common weight loss procedure performed. The complications of RYGB are diverse and vary based on the specific technique used. Some complications are relatively specific to the surgical approach (open versus laparoscopic). Certain complications are seen during the early postoperative period, while others may become present weeks to months after the surgery.

12.7.1.1 Leaks
A gastrointestinal leak is one of the most dreaded complications in patients who undergo gastric bypass for morbid obesity. The incidence of anastomotic leakage after LRYGB ranges from 0 to 5.2 % and can be as high as 13 % in revision surgery, especially after converting a failed vertical banded gastroplasty to an RYGB. Anastomotic leaks remain the second leading cause of death following LRYGB (causing 6–17 % of the mortality). The mortality rate is higher for jejunojejunal leaks than gastrojejunal leaks. However, most leaks occur at the site of gastrojejunostomy or on the staple line of the gastric pouch. If not diagnosed in a timely manner, the mortality rate can be as high as 17 %. The timing of leaks has a biphasic distribution. Early leaks associated with technical problems occur within 24–48 h after surgery. Late leaks that occur 5–10 days postoperatively may be related to ischemia or poor healing of the anastomosis.

The risk factors for developing leaks are super obesity (BMI > 50), male sex, age > 65 years old, having multiple comorbidities, and patients undergoing revision surgery. However, the primary causes of leaks are the technical factors

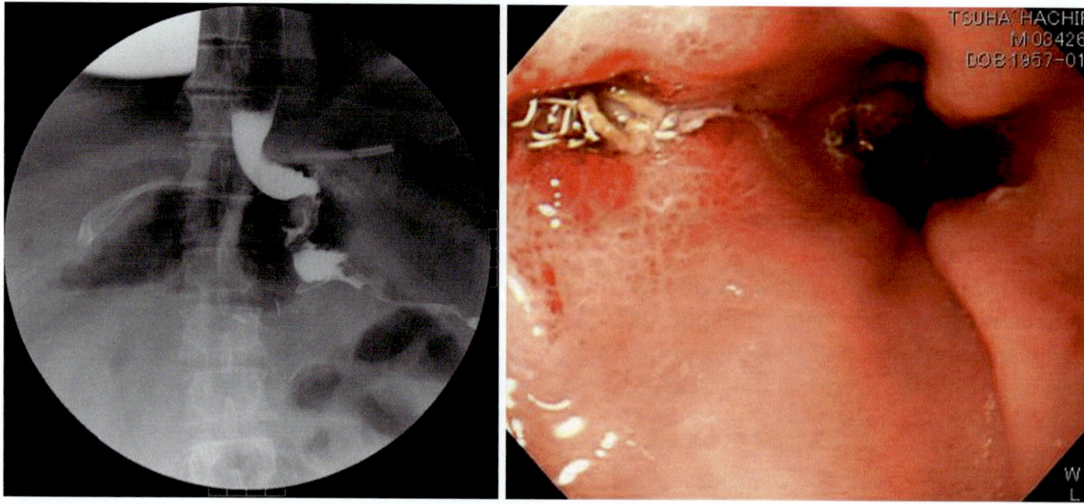

Fig. 12.1 Leak from gastric pouch

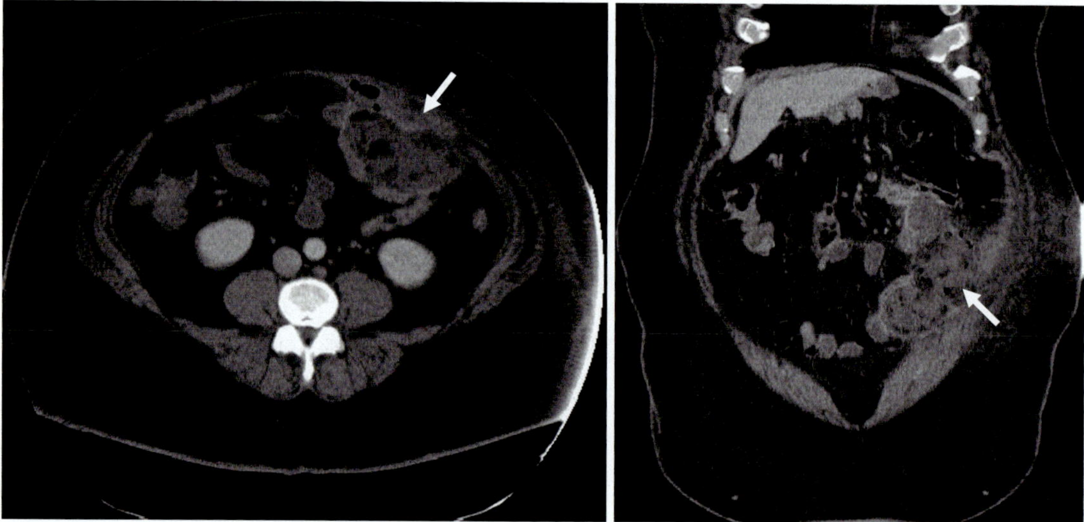

Fig. 12.2 Abscess (*arrow*) formation due to leak from jejunojejunal anastomosis

during surgery such as excessive tension, an inadequate blood supply to the anastomotic site following insufficient oxygenation, and subsequent ischemia.

The early clinical signs of a leak are a low-grade fever, respiratory compromise, or unexplained tachycardia (>120 bpm), tachypnea, hypoxia, and extreme anxiety. These signs may also be present in the setting of a pulmonary embolism. It is not rare for peritoneal irritation to be lacking in bariatric patients under such an emergency condition.

Leaks may be radiographically confirmed by a water-soluble contrast swallow (Fig. 12.1) or contrast abdominal computed tomographic (CT) scan (Fig. 12.2). These may be identified on the studies as an oral contrast extravasation from the anastomosis, extraluminal air or fluid collections adjacent to the gastric pouch, or as diffuse ascites. If leaks are suspected clinically, especially in patients with hemodynamic instability, emergency surgical exploration should be performed even if the imaging studies are negative. Multiple studies have shown that re-exploration is safer compared to missing or delaying the treatment of a leak. Surgical exploration and the management of leaks are often feasible via a laparoscopic approach.

The surgical principles for treating a leak include broad-spectrum antibiotic coverage, identification and repair of the defect, irrigation and control of the contaminated area, and making access for feeding (jejunostomy or gastrostomy tube). With leaks at the gastrojejunal anastomosis, if the condition of the tissues is not bad, the defect may be closed with primary suturing, followed by irrigation of the area and the placement of drains. When primary closure of the defect is not possible, wide drainage is an option.

Jejunojejunostomy leaks are a serious complication, with a higher mortality rate compared to other leaks of up to 40 %. Surgical intervention must be promptly performed due to the presence of hemodynamic instability or rapid clinical deterioration. In general, these anastomotic defects can be more easily detected and repaired than those of the gastrojejunostomy. It is recommended that decompression of the excluded stomach using tubing gastrostomy in patients with complicated conditions.

Surgical therapies for persistent leaks are technically difficult and often unsuccessful. New approaches using endoscopic repair techniques include the use of fibrin glue and/or placement of covered stents and have been shown to be safe and effective in some patients.

12.7.1.2 Acute Gastric Remnant Dilatation

Gastric remnant dilatation is a rare (0.6 %) but potentially lethal complication following Roux-en-Y gastric bypass. The gastric remnant is a blind pouch and may become distended due to the closed-loop obstruction that can develop following obstruction of the biliopancreatic limb or paralytic ileus. Progressive distension can ultimately lead to a blowout of the staple line, spillage of massive gastric contents, and subsequent severe peritonitis.

The clinical features of this complication include severe epigastric pain, hiccups, left upper quadrant tympany, shoulder pain, abdominal distension, tachycardia, or shortness of breath. Radiographic assessment may demonstrate a large gastric bubble on a plain abdominal x-ray or CT scan (Fig. 12.3). The treatment of this consists of percutaneous gastrostomy or emergency surgical decomtpression with a gastrostomy. Immediate surgical exploration and decompression are required if percutaneous drainage is not

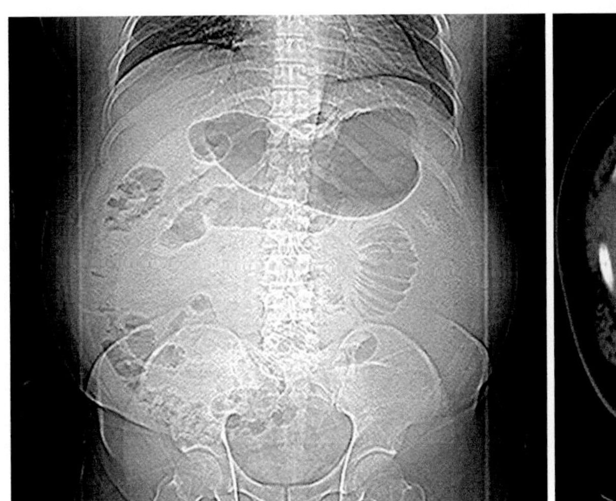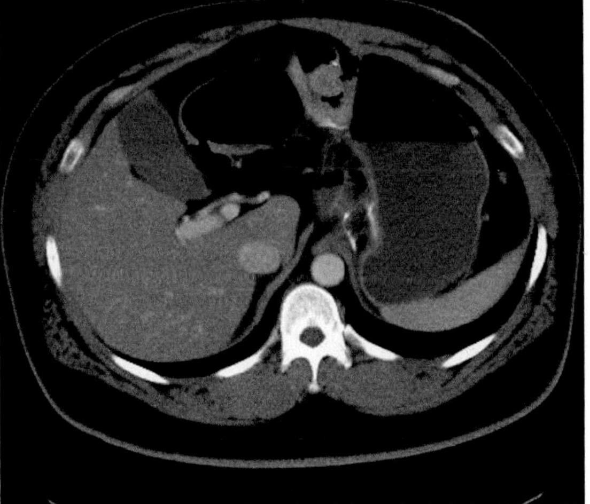

Fig. 12.3 Acute gastric dilatation

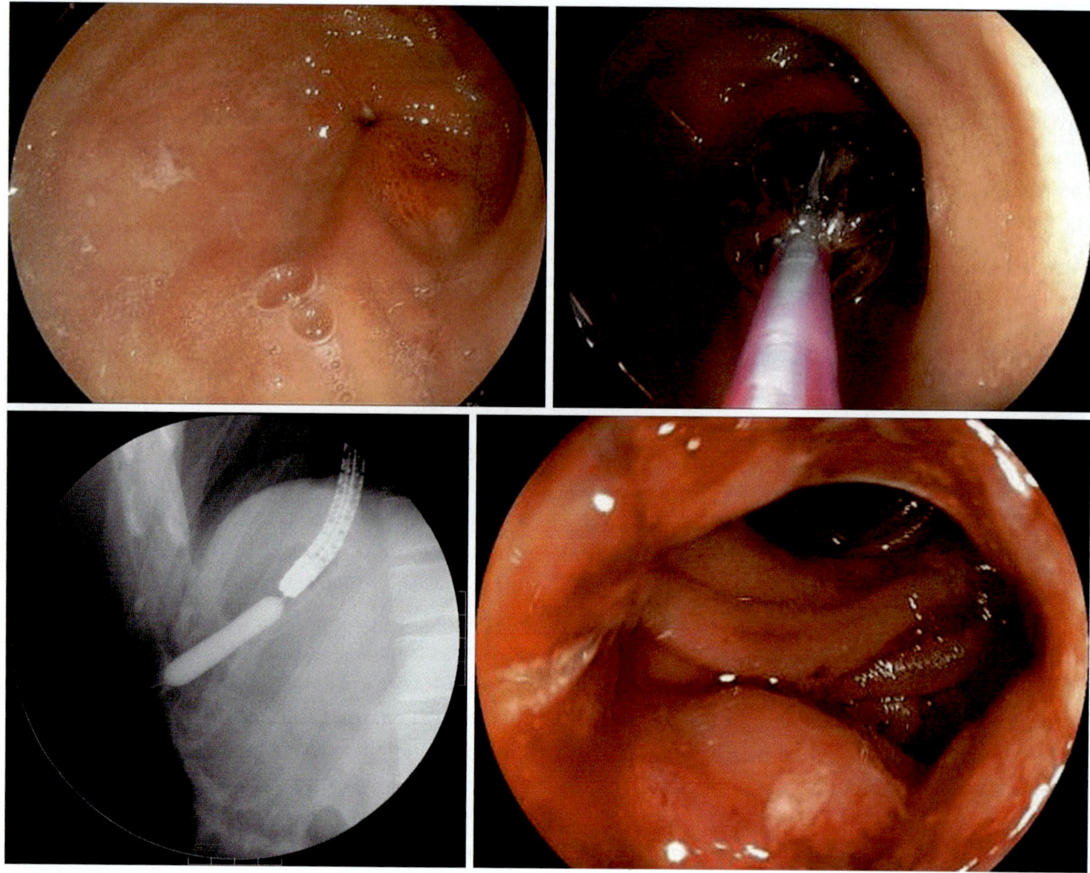

Fig. 12.4 Endoscopic balloon dilation for stomal stenosis

feasible or if a perforation is suspected. It also requires the appropriate management of the underlying biliary limb obstruction.

12.7.1.3 Stomal Stenosis

Stomal (anastomotic) stenosis has been described in 6–20 % of patients who have undergone RYGB. The etiology is uncertain, although tissue ischemia or increased tension on the gastrojejunal anastomosis is believed to have a role. The stomal stenosis rate is higher in LRYGB and may be related to the use of the small-diameter circular staplers, which are commonly used by many surgeons.

Patients typically present several weeks after surgery with nausea, vomiting, dysphagia, gastroesophageal reflux, and eventually an inability to tolerate the oral intake of foods or liquids. The diagnosis is usually established by endoscopy or with an upper gastrointestinal series. Endoscopic balloon dilation is usually successful (Fig. 12.4). Repeat dilation sessions may be required for

some patients. Surgical revision is reserved for those who have persistent stenosis despite repeated dilations.

12.7.1.4 Marginal Ulcers

Marginal ulcers have been reported in up to 16 % of patients after RYGB. Ulcers can occur from several weeks to many years after surgery. Marginal ulcers occur near the gastrojejunostomy and result from acid injuring the jejunum, or they can be associated with a gastrogastric fistula. The risk factors for marginal ulcers include a large proximal gastric pouch; poor tissue perfusion due to tension or ischemia at the anastomosis; the presence of foreign material, such as staples or nonabsorbable sutures; excess acid exposure in the gastric pouch due to gastrogastric fistulas; the use of nonsteroidal anti-inflammatory drugs (NSAIDs); *Helicobacter pylori* infection; or smoking.

Patients with marginal ulcers present with nausea, heartburn, epigastric pain, gastrointesti-

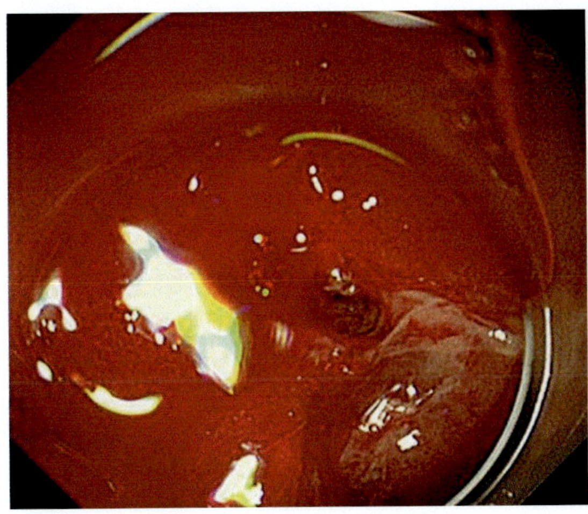
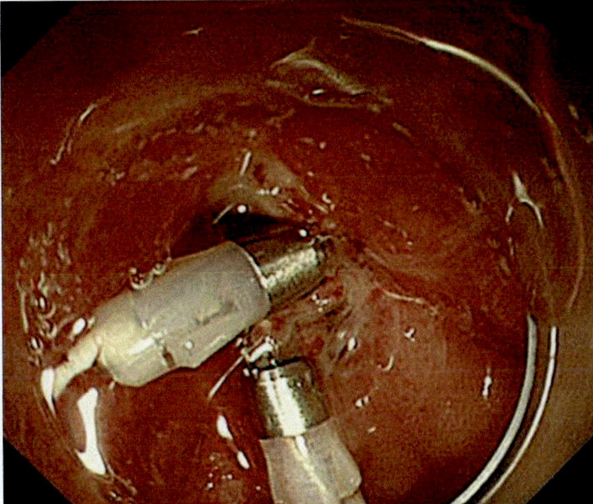

Fig. 12.5 Acute bleeding from marginal ulcer

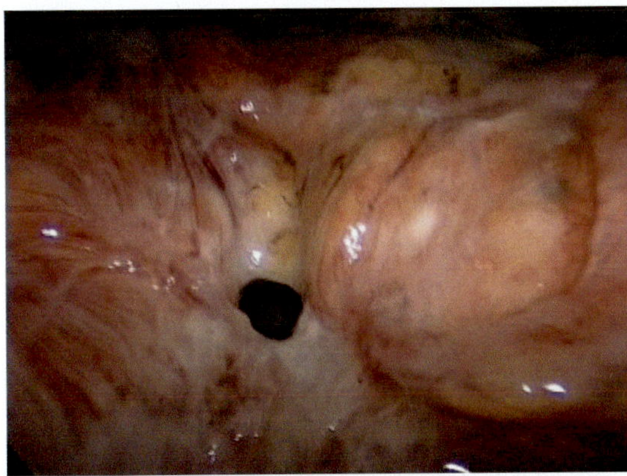

Fig. 12.6 Acute perforation

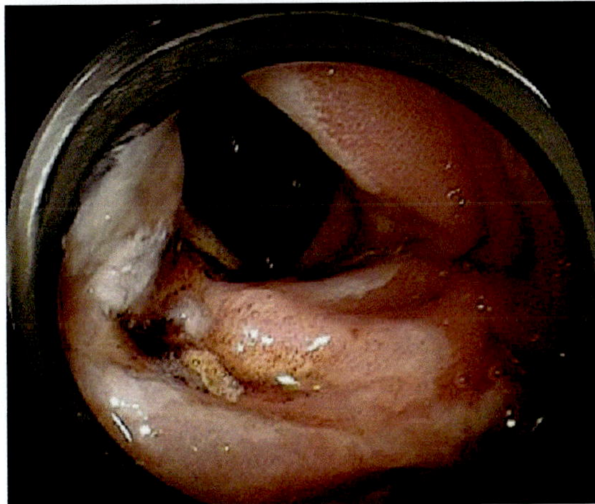

Fig. 12.7 Marginal ulcer

nal (GI) bleeding, and/or perforation (Figs. 12.5 and 12.6). The diagnosis of a marginal ulcer is established by upper endoscopy (Fig. 12.7). The majority of patients (95 %) can be successfully treated by medical treatment consisting of gastric acid suppression, such as using proton pump inhibitors. In addition, NSAIDS should be discontinued, and patients should be encouraged to stop smoking.

After maximal medical management fails, if persistent symptoms and signs of ulcers are present, this is an indication that surgery is necessary and can include resection of the anastomosis and making a smaller gastric pouch. Perforated ulcers with generalized peritonitis and upper GI bleeding that cannot be controlled by endoscopic therapy also need emergency surgery.

12.7.1.5 Gastrogastric Fistulas

A gastrogastric fistula (GGF) results from a recanalization between the gastric pouch and excluded distal gastric remnant, despite the fact that the stomach has been divided using stapler devices. The incidence of the complication varies in literature from 2 to 25 %. GGF does not require urgent intervention, but it can lead to three major long-term problems: recurrent stomal ulcers, gastroesophageal reflux, and sudden weight regain. The presence of these complications should prompt an evaluation for GGF. They can be detected easily by an upper gastrointestinal series. Endoscopy can also detect this condition (Fig. 12.8), though small fistulas may be difficult to identify. In patients who have suboptimal weight loss or refractory ulcers, surgical re-separation of the

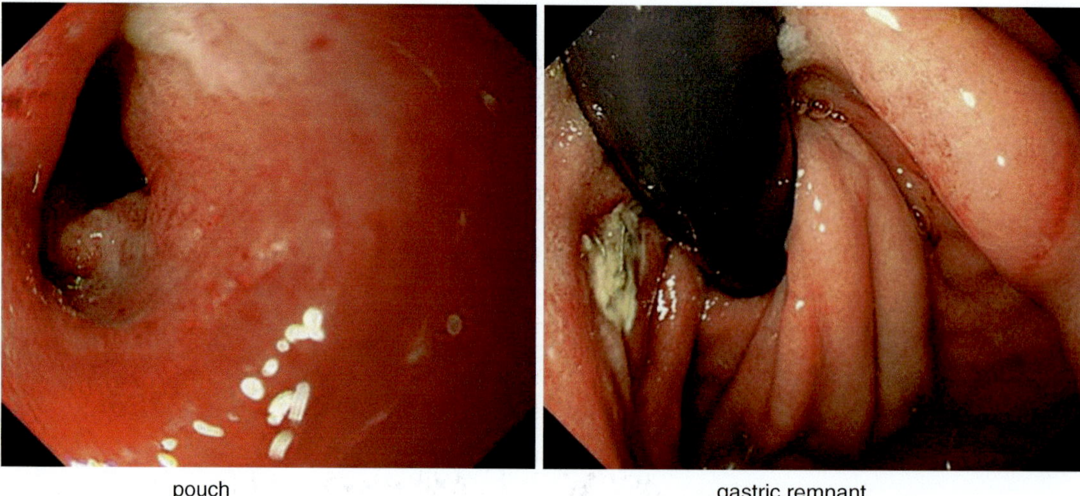

Fig. 12.8 Gastrogastric fistula

gastric pouch and excluded stomach may be necessary. Treatment with an endoluminal technique may be possible in the future.

12.7.1.6 Internal Hernias and Small Bowel Obstructions

Small bowel obstruction can occur through several mechanisms, both early and late after RYGB. Adhesive bowel obstructions can occur after both open and laparoscopic approaches (Fig. 12.9). Internal hernias are the most common cause of postoperative obstruction following laparoscopic Roux-en-Y gastric bypass. This is because the Roux-en-Y anatomy is associated with potential internal spaces through which herniation of the small intestine can occur. Three potential areas of internal herniation are the mesenteric defect at the jejunojejunostomy, the space between the transverse mesocolon and Roux limb mesentery (Petersen's space), and the defect in the transverse mesocolon if the Roux limb is passed retrocolically. Internal hernias have been described in 0–5 % of patients undergoing laparoscopic bariatric surgery. Hernias through the transverse mesocolon are the most common and require surgical intervention.

To reduce the incidence of internal hernias, all areas of potential herniation should be closed with nonabsorbable sutures. Radiological evaluations may be useful, with CT scans providing

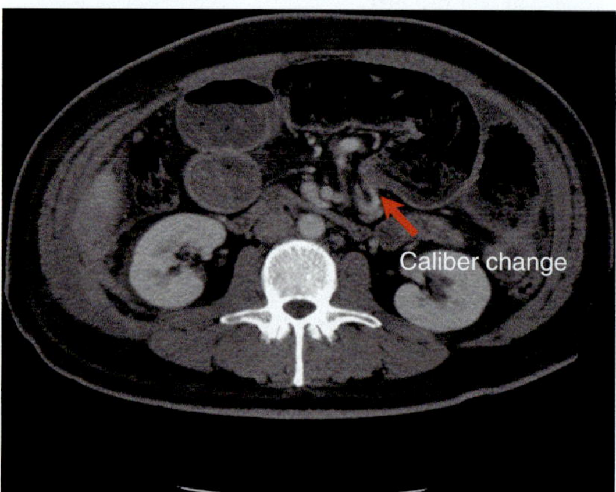

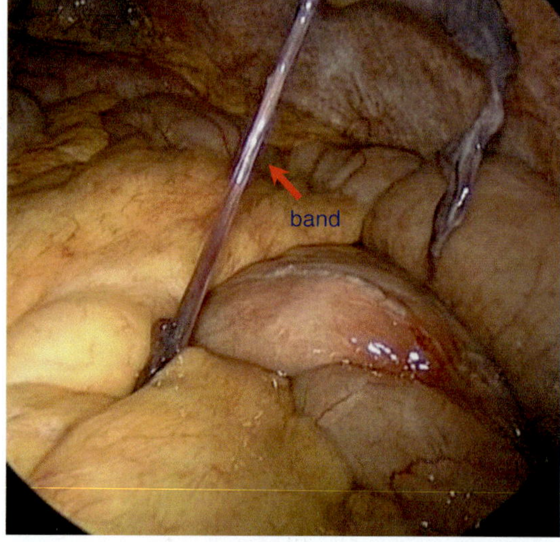

Fig. 12.9 Small bowel obstruction due to band formation

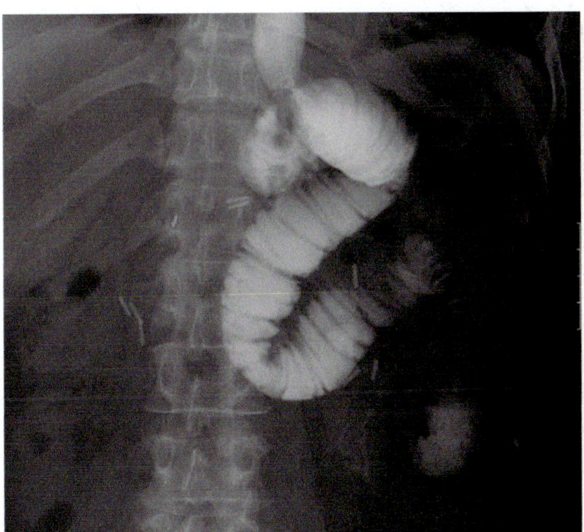
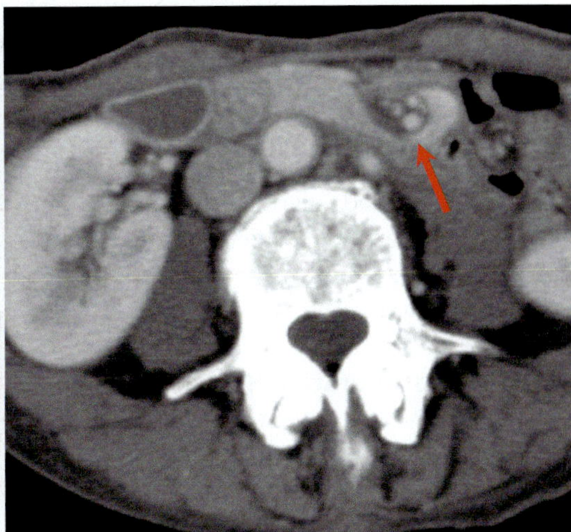

Fig. 12.10 Petersen's hernia. Mesenteric swirl sign (*arrow*)

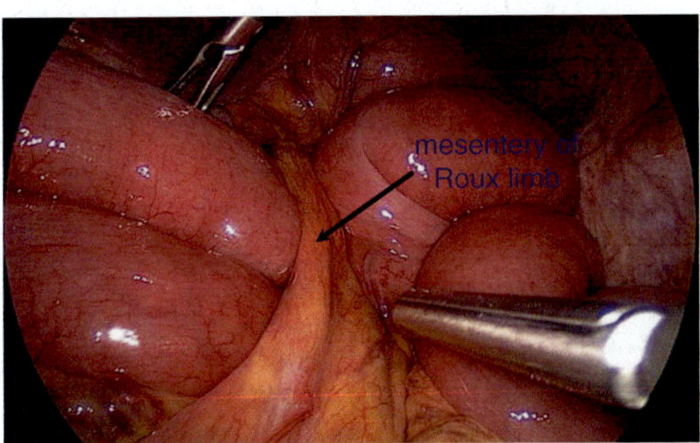

Fig. 12.11 Petersen's hernia

the most accurate diagnostic tool for internal hernias. The "mesenteric swirl sign," which indicates mesenteric vascular twisting on a CT scan, is the best indicator of an internal hernia following gastric bypass (Fig. 12.10). A patient suspected to have an internal hernia as the etiology of their abdominal pain indicates urgent surgical exploration. The treatment of internal hernias can be done laparoscopically (Fig. 12.11). The exploration begins at the gastrojejunostomy, and the entire small bowel should be checked to the cecum, including the jejunojejunal anastomosis, biliopancreatic limb, and remnant stomach, with all potential mesenteric defects inspected. If an internal hernia was present, after the reduction of an internal hernia, all remaining mesenteric defects should be closed with nonabsorbable running sutures. If exploration is performed in a timely manner, the rate of bowel resection is relatively low.

However, strangulated hernias may require extensive small bowel resection and can potentially result in the development of short bowel syndrome. Therefore, if an internal hernia with bowel ischemia is suspected, then surgical exploration should be performed promptly without hesitation.

12.7.1.7 Cholelithiasis

Rapid weight loss can be a risk factor for the development of gallstones. Cholelithiasis develops in as many as 38 % of patients within 6 months of bariatric surgery, and 10–41 % of such patients become symptomatic. The high frequency of cholelithiasis can be reduced to as low as 2 % with a 6-month course of ursodeoxycholic acid (UDCA), given prophylactically after weight loss surgery.

The decision to perform a cholecystectomy at the time of bypass is controversial. There is no evidence that simultaneous cholecystectomy for gallstones at the time of RYGB benefits the patients. Cholecystectomy can be performed safely on those who develop cholelithiasis. However, choledocholithiasis may be more difficult to manage after performing gastric bypass surgery.

12.7.1.8 Dumping Syndrome

Dumping syndrome can occur in up to 50 % of post-gastric bypass patients when high levels of simple carbohydrates are ingested. Although sometimes considered a complication of gastric bypass, in most cases, dumping syndrome is considered to contribute to weight loss, in part by causing the patient to modify his/her eating habits. The lightheadedness, dizziness, abdominal pain, bloating, and diarrhea associated with dumping syndrome are often potent negative reinforcements promoting the loss of desire for concentrated sweets.

12.7.1.9 Postoperative Hypoglycemia

A small number of patients develop blackouts and seizures after weight loss surgery due to a severe form of recurrent hyperinsulinemic hypoglycemia. Pancreatic nesidioblastosis has been proposed as a mechanism for the pathological finding of beta islet hypertrophy in these patients, although a few cases of insulinomas have been found. Gastric bypass-induced weight loss may also unmask an underlying beta-cell defect or contribute to pathological islet hyperplasia.

12.7.1.10 Vitamin, Mineral, and Nutritional Deficiencies

Vitamin, mineral, and nutritional deficiencies are common in severely obese patients and can be exacerbated following bariatric surgery, making postoperative, lifelong compliance with appropriate dietary choices and vitamin supplementation imperative. After RYGB, decreased oral intake, as well as altered absorption of food from the stomach and small bowel, reduces the absorption of various micronutrients, particularly iron, calcium, vitamin B12, thiamine, and folate. Nutritional deficiencies are expected following bariatric surgery, and supplementation is the best form of prevention.

12.7.2 Laparoscopic Sleeve Gastrectomy

The number of LSG operations has been rising. This new procedure is not only a simple, restrictive procedure without anastomosis but is also effective as a sole weight loss surgery. Though this is a simple procedure, simple does not mean easy and safe. There are troublesome

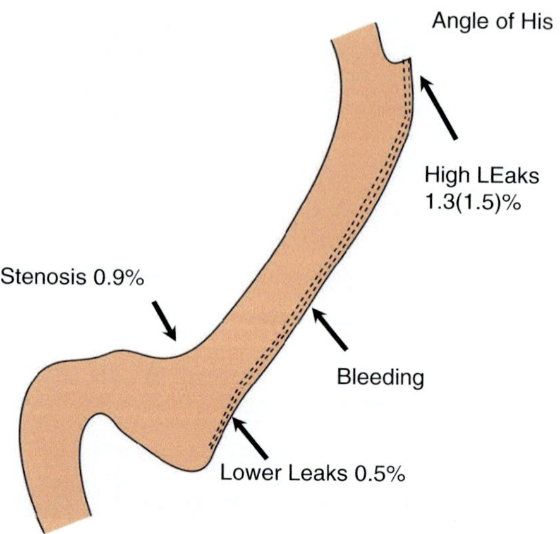

Fig. 12.12 Critical point of leak and stenosis of sleeve gastrectomy

complications that are not seen in other bariatric procedures after LSG. It is important to learn prevention and management of these complications.

The most common postoperative complications of LSG include bleeding, narrowing or stenosis of the sleeve, and prolonged leaks (Fig. 12.12).

12.7.2.1 Bleeding

Bleeding can occur from the gastroepiploic, short gastric vessels or from the spleen during the dissection of the greater curvature. Most bleeding problems associated with LSG occur from the staple line after the transection of the stomach. The bleeding is most likely a result of the large staples used for the thick tissue in the distal stomach. Large staples are not adequate to seal small vessels. This has led many surgeons to reinforce the staple line by over-sewing, buttressing, or both. These reinforcements of the staple line have reduced the amount of bleeding from the gastric transection line (Fig. 12.13). However, such reinforcements are cost- and time-consuming.

12.7.2.2 Stenosis

Narrowing or stenosis can create gastric outlet obstruction. The presentation varies depending on the severity of the obstruction but can include dysphagia, vomiting, dehydration, and

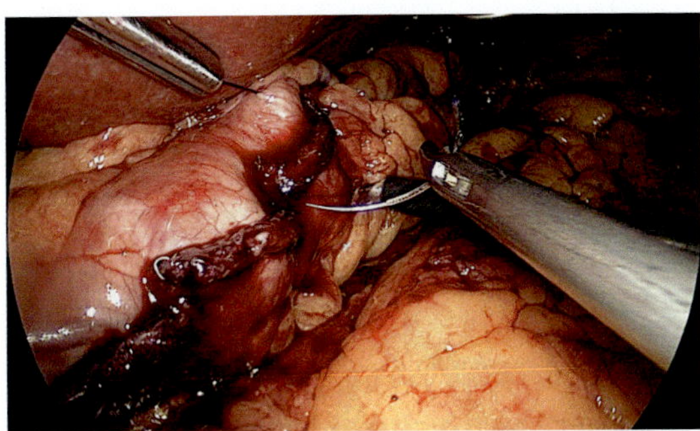

Fig. 12.13 Reinforcements of staple line

the inability to tolerate an oral diet. The gastro-esophageal junction and the incisura angularis are the two most common areas where stenosis occurs and can be diagnosed by an upper gastrointestinal series and endoscopy (Fig. 12.14). Sleeve stenosis, which is sometimes difficult to recognize, can lead to a fistula remaining open. Even if the endoscope passes through the sleeve, it does not mean that a stenosis does not exist, because there can be a spiral sleeve.

The most common reasons for the development of narrowing or stenosis are due to stapling issues. The reasons of sleeve stenosis are firing linear staplers too close bougie, over-sewing the

staple line, and using a bougie that is too small. The preferred bougie size is currently being debated in the literature and can range from 30 to 60 French. In most cases, surgeons use a 36–40 French bougie for the sleeve construction. Twist gastric sleeve and spiral gastric sleeve can be sleeve obstruction.

The first line of treatment for stenosis is endoscopic pneumatic dilation. If the area of stenosis is too long, surgical intervention may be necessary with gastric stricturoplasty (seromyotomy), conversion to a LRYGB or total gastrectomy.

12.7.2.3 Sleeve Leaks

Sleeve leaks after LSG are one of the most dreaded complications, reported in 1–7 % of patients. The early clinical signs of leaks are epigastric pain, left shoulder tip pain, low-grade fever, respiratory compromise, unexplained tachycardia (>120 bpm), tachypnea, hypoxia, and extreme anxiety. It is not rare for peritoneal irritation to be lacking in bariatric patients, even under emergency conditions.

Leaks may be radiographically confirmed by a water-soluble contrast swallow or contrast-enhanced abdominal CT scan. The leaks may be identified on the studies as an oral contrast

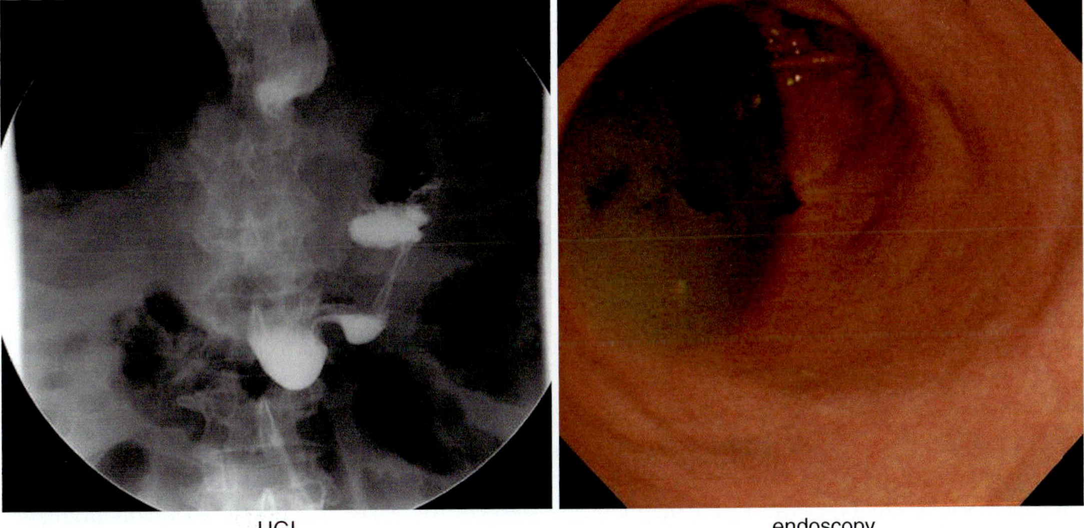

Fig. 12.14 Sleeve stenosis

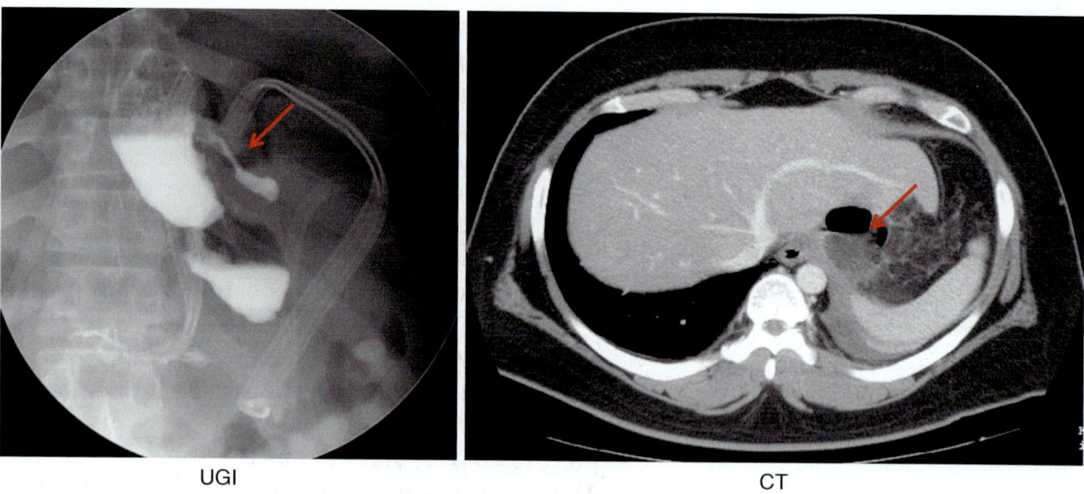

Fig. 12.15 Sleeve leaks (*arrows*)

extravasation from the long staple line, extraluminal air or fluid collections adjacent to the gastric sleeve (Fig. 12.15).

There are two common sites of leaks that have been known after LSG. One is at the end of the staple line of the gastric antrum (low leak), and the other is at the end of the staple line near the esophagogastric junction (high leak) (Fig. 12.12). The causes of leaks at the angle of His include using a bougie that was too small, poor blood supply, physiological obstruction by the pylorus, mechanical obstruction by an L-shaped sleeve, negative pressure from the thorax, no remnant stomach to block the fistula, and long tortuous fistula tracts.

To prevent leaks, it is necessary to ensure that the sleeve is not too tight, that the stapler is fired lateral to the angle of His, and that an intraoperative leak test is performed selectively. Most leaks are due to local factors at the site of the staple line, such as an inadequate blood supply and oxygenation, which impede the healing process. Although the blood supply to the stomach is usually robust, the gastroesophageal junction tends to be an area of decreased vascularity and thus is more prone to leaks. Additionally, the stomach tends to be thinner at the angle of His, and some authors of medical papers suggest that the large staple height used by many surgeons may not adequately seal this area of the stomach. Some surgeons recommend leaving a small portion of stomach distal to the angle of His and then imbricating this with a running silk suture. However, clinical studies have not provided evidence that reinforcing the suture line decreases the rate of leaks after sleeve gastrectomy. Sleeve gastrectomy produces a high intragastric pressure, which can affect the healing process and lengthen the amount of time required for a leak to close.

Reoperation with primary repair during the early postoperative course (<POD 2) is the best option for a leak that develops after LSG. Clinically stable patients may be able to undergo ultrasound- or CT-guided percutaneous drainage, antibiotic therapy, and parenteral nutrition or nasoenteral feeding until the leak is healed. Endoscopic injection of fibrin glue and the use of self-expanding coated stents have also been employed for the management of leaks (Fig. 12.16), but a stent should not be used for a distal leak because of the possibility of migration. If a stent is left in place too long, it can become very difficult to remove.

If the leaks may be prolonged by the treatment described above, definitive surgery, such as total gastrectomy or Roux-jejunal loop anastomosis to the persistent fistula, has been reported as a last resort. An early diagnosis, adequate drainage, and gastric decompression are the mainstay of treatment for leaks.

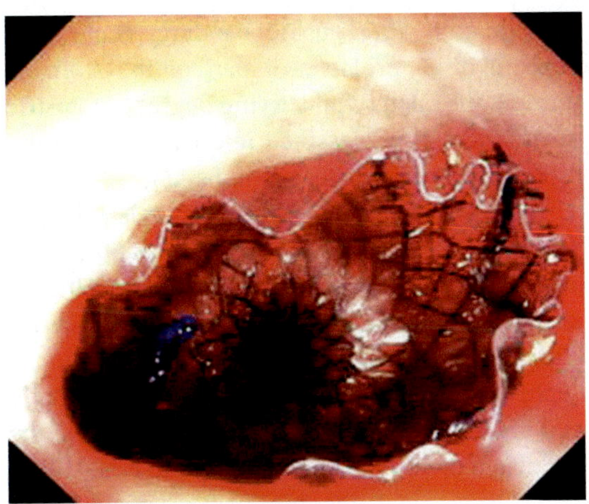

Fig. 12.16 Self-expanding coated stent

12.7.2.4 Gastroesophageal Reflux Disease (GERD)

Gastroesophageal reflux after LSG presents with classic symptoms, such as burning pain, heart burn, and regurgitation. It can occur as an early or late complication. The first line of treatment is anti-reflux medical therapy. GERD unresponsive to anti-reflux medical therapy with no clear anatomical abnormalities, such as stoma stenosis or a hiatal hernia, can be effectively treated by conversion to LRYGB.

12.7.3 Laparoscopic Adjustable Gastric Banding

LAGB was the third most common weight loss surgery performed worldwide in 2011 and has the lowest mortality rate among all bariatric procedures. However, LAGB is associated with several complications. An initial trial of LAGB in the Unites States showed disappointing weight loss outcomes and high complication rates, associated with relatively high revision surgery rates (40 %). Following changes in the surgical technique, subsequent trials in Europe, Australia, and the United States have shown fewer complications. Nevertheless, the long-term results from a series of 78 LAGB patients showed that nearly 40 % of patients experienced major complications, which included pouch dilatation (11 %),

band erosion (28 %), and band infection (1 %). Minor complications included incisional hernias (5 %), port-tubing disconnections (20 %), and port infections (2 %).

Both early and late complications of LAGB can occur. The early complications include acute stomal obstruction, band infection, gastric perforation, hemorrhage, bronchopneumonia, delayed gastric emptying, and pulmonary embolism. Pulmonary embolism was the most common cause of early mortality in a series of LAGB patients. The late complications include band erosion, band slippage or prolapse, port or tubing malfunction, leakage at the port site tubing or band, pouch or esophageal dilatation, and esophagitis. Almost 50 % of all patients will need surgical revision or removal of the band. Failed bands can generally be converted to other bariatric procedures, such as RYGB or duodenal switch.

In addition, the rate of long-term complications and rates of reoperation are higher with LAGB compared with RYGB. In a prospective study of 442 patients matched for age, gender, and BMI, patients undergoing LAGB had a significantly higher rate of long-term complications compared with patients undergoing LRYGB.

12.7.3.1 Stomal Obstruction

Stomal obstruction is defined as an obstruction of the passage of food from the gastric pouch to the rest of the stomach. Acute stomal obstruction is an early complication that can occur in up to 14 % of LAGB patients. Patients usually present with persistent nausea, vomiting, sialorrhea, and an inability to swallow or have oral intake.

The diagnosis is confirmed with an upper gastrointestinal series demonstrating no passage of contrast beyond the band.

Acute stomal obstruction due to edema can initially be treated conservatively with nasogastric tube decompression until the edema subsides, although the potential for aspiration pneumonia and stomach ischemia exists. Persistent obstruction requires surgical revision or removal of the band.

12.7.3.2 Port Infection

Port infection has been reported in 0.3–9 % of LAGB patients. Because the port is a foreign

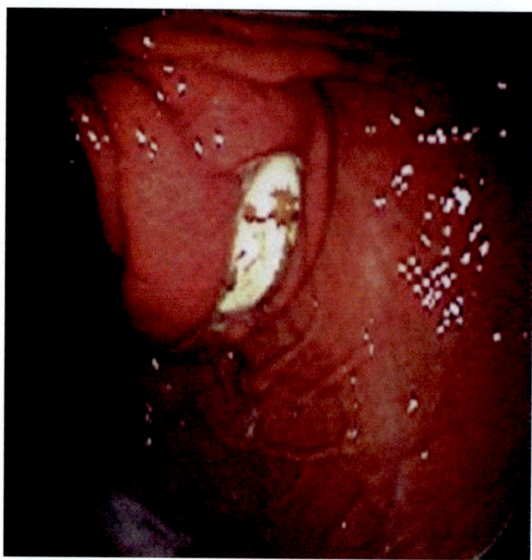

Fig. 12.17 Band erosion

body, port infection is treated with surgical removal, especially in association with band erosion.

12.7.3.3 Band Erosion

Band erosion is defined as the partial or complete movement of a synthetic band into the gastric lumen of the stomach. It has been reported in 1–7 % of LAGB patients, and it is thought to occur as a result of gastric wall ischemia from an excessively tight band. Band erosion is a late complication and occurs at a mean of 22 months after surgery.

Most symptoms of erosion are of a benign nature, non-urgent and non-life-threatening. The clinical signs of band erosion include infection, failure of weight loss, and/or nausea and vomiting. Band erosion can be diagnosed by endoscopy, and the treatment involves removal of the band, which can be done laparoscopically (Fig. 12.17).

12.7.3.4 Band Slippage and Gastric Prolapse

After LAGB, the surface of the stomach can slip acutely through the band, associated with an episode of severe vomiting. This is called band slippage and is a relatively common postoperative complication after gastric banding. Band slippage involves prolapse of part of the stomach through the band, with varying degrees of gastric obstruction. It is classified into two types: anterior slippage and posterior slippage.

Anterior slippage involves the migration of the band in the cephalad direction, which creates an acute angle with the stomach pouch and esophagus, resulting in obstruction. Posterior slippage occurs when the stomach migrates in the cephalad direction, displacing the band caudally and creating a new pouch. In recent studies, the incidence of slippage was reported to be 2–14 %. The perigastric technique was associated with frequent gastric prolapse. However, the newer pars flaccida technique has significantly decreased the incidence of this complication.

Gastric prolapse is characterized by food intolerance, epigastric pain, and acid reflux. The diagnosis is confirmed with an upper gastrointestinal series demonstrating either malposition of the band or dilatation and prolapse of the gastric pouch (Fig. 12.18). Depending on the presentation, surgery may be required urgently. Repair of the prolapse can sometimes be accomplished by repositioning the band, but often the band needs to be replaced or removed altogether, especially if inflammation is present.

12.7.3.5 Esophagitis

Esophagitis and reflux are infrequent following LAGB. Deflation of the band and acid-suppression therapy are the most common forms of treatment. However, if they are intractable to medical therapy, band removal or conversion to another procedure, such as LRYGB, may be necessary.

12.7.3.6 Esophageal and Gastric Pouch Dilatation

Esophageal and gastric pouch dilatation proximal to the band device without slippage has been observed in as many as 10 % of patients. This so-called pseudoachalasia syndrome may develop when the band is excessively inflated or in cases of excessive amounts of food intake. Pouch dilatation has also been associated with a history of binge eating behavior. Patients often present with

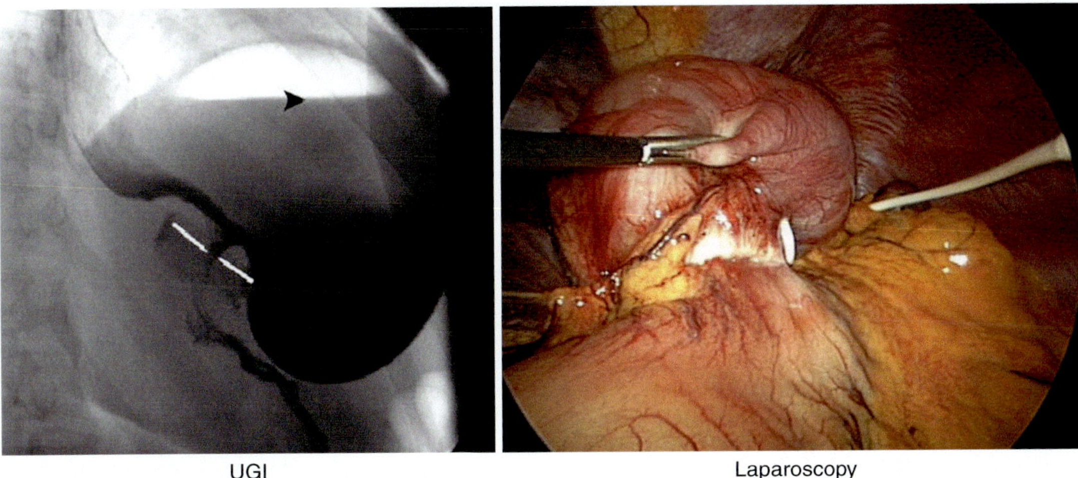

UGI   Laparoscopy

Fig. 12.18 Band slippage. *Black arrow head* air fluid level; *white line* constriction due to slippage

food and saliva intolerance, reflux, and epigastric discomfort. The diagnosis can be confirmed with an upper gastrointestinal series.

The initial treatment should be removal of all the fluid from the band and behavioral diet modifications. However, persistent dilatation may require replacement of the band in a new location on the stomach or conversion to a different procedure.

12.7.3.7 Hiatus Hernia

Hiatus hernia is often a preexisting but unrecognized condition in patients undergoing bariatric surgery. This can lead to ongoing intractable reflux necessitating reoperation or band removal. A simple crural repair can be performed at the initial operation to avoid these complications.

12.7.4 Biliopancreatic Diversion and Duodenal Switch

Early complications and the management of biliopancreatic diversion and duodenal switch (BPD/DS) are similar to that of LRYGB. Both BPD and DS are mainly malabsorptive procedures that rely on limiting the absorption of lipids and essential fatty acids to a relatively short segment of the small intestine (50–100 cm), as well as on decreasing the gastric reservoir size. BPD/DS has not become widespread because of the technical complexity of the procedure, with relatively high surgical morbidity and mortality (1.1 %) rates. In addition, long-term nutritional outcomes, including dehydration, calorie malnutrition, hypoproteinemia, anemia, metabolic bone disease, and deficiencies of vitamins, are of concern. These complications regarding nutrition can almost always be prevented with supplementation and monitoring. For this reason, it is important for lifelong follow-ups after BPD/DS as among other weight loss surgeries.

Further Videos

Electronic supplementary material is available in the online version of this chapter at (doi:10.1007/978-3-642-35591-2_12) and accessible for authorised users. Videos can also be accessed at http://www.springerimages.com/videos/978-3-642-35590-5

References

1. Buchwald H, Oien DM. Metabolic/bariatric surgery worldwide 2011. Obes Surg. 2013;23(4):427.
2. Buchwald H, Avidor Y, et al. Bariatric surgery: a systemic review and analysis. JAMA. 2004;292(14):1724.
3. Longitudinal Assessment of Bariatric Surgery Consortium. Perioperative safety in the longitudinal assessment of bariatric surgery. N Engl J Med. 2009;36(5):445.

 4. Maggard MA, Shugamann LR, et al. Meta-analysis: surgical treatment of obesity. Ann Intern Med. 2005;142(7):547.
 5. Buchwald H, Esok R. Trends in mortality in bariatric surgery: asystemic review and meta-analysis. Surgery. 2007;142(4):621.
 6. Lancaster RH, Hutter MM. Bands and bypass: 30-day morbidity and mortality of bariatric surgical procedures assessment by prospective, multi-center, risk-adjusted ACS-NSQIP data. Surg Endosc. 2008;22(12):2554.
 7. Schauer P, Ikramuddin S, Hamad G, Gourash W. The learning curve for laparoscopic Roux-en-Y gastric bypass is 100 cases. Surg Endosc. 2003;17:212.
 8. Wittgrove AC, Clark GW. Laparoscopic gastric bypass, Roux-en-Y-500 patients: technique and results, with 3–60 month follow-up. Obes Surg. 2000;10:233.
 9. Nguyen NT, Goldman C, Rosenquist CJ, et al. Laparoscopic versus open gastric bypass: a randomized study of outcomes, quality of life, and costs. Ann Surg. 2001;234:279.
10. Higa KD, Boone KB, Ho T. Complications of the laparoscopic Roux-en-Y gastric bypass: 1,040 patients – what have we learned? Obes Surg. 2000;10:509.
11. Shikora SA, Kim JJ, Tarnoff ME. Comparison of permanent and nonpermanent staple line buttressing materials for linear gastric staple lines during laparoscopic Roux-en-Y gastric bypass. Surg Obes Relat Dis. 2008;4:729.
12. Fukumoto R, Orlina J, McGinty J, Teixeira J. Use of Polyflex stents in treatment of acute esophageal and gastric leaks after bariatric surgery. Surg Obes Relat Dis. 2007;3:68.
13. Morino M, Toppino M, Forestieri P, et al. Mortality after bariatric surgery: analysis of 13,871 morbidly obese patients from a national registry. Ann Surg. 2007;246:1002.
14. Capella JF, Capella RF. Gastro-gastric fistulas and marginal ulcers in gastric bypass procedures for weight reduction. Obes Surg. 1999;9:22.
15. Eisendrath P, Cremer M, Himpens J, et al. Endotherapy including temporary stenting of fistulas of the upper gastrointestinal tract after laparoscopic bariatric surgery. Endoscopy. 2007;39:625.
16. Himpens J, Cadière GB, Bazi M, et al. Long-term outcomes of laparoscopic adjustable gastric banding. Arch Surg. 2011;146:802.
17. Chevallier JM, Zinzindohoué F, Douard R, et al. Complications after laparoscopic adjustable gastric banding for morbid obesity: experience with 1,000 patients over 7 years. Obes Surg. 2004;14:407.
18. Gagner M, Deitel M, Kalberer TL, et al. The second international consensus summit for sleeve gastrectomy, March 19–21, 2009. Surg Obes Relat Dis. 2009;5:476.
19. Deitel M, et al. Third international summit: current status of sleeve gastrectomy. Surg Obes Relat Dis. 2011;7(6):749–59.
20. Oshiro T, Kasama K, Umezawa A, et al. Successful management of refractory staple line leakage at the esophagogastric junction after a sleeve gastrectomy using the HANAROSTENT. Obes Surg. 2010;20:530.
21. Serra C, Baltasar A, Andreo L, et al. Treatment of gastric leaks with coated self-expanding stents after sleeve gastrectomy. Obes Surg. 2007;17:866.